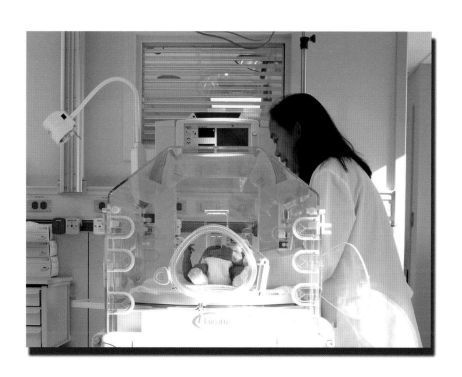

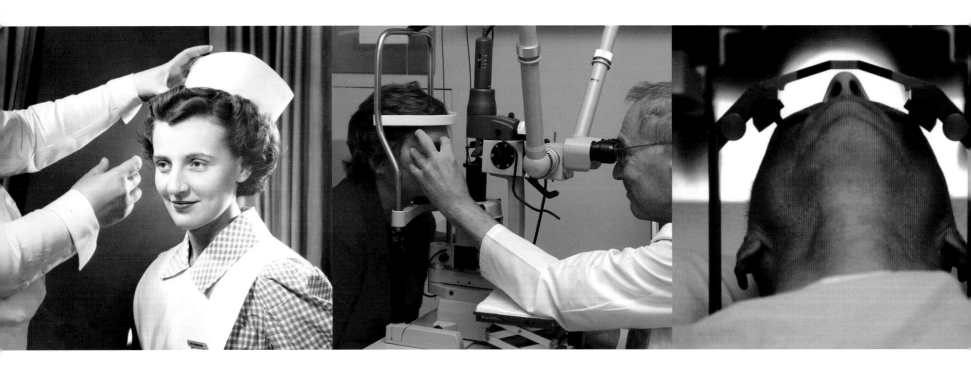

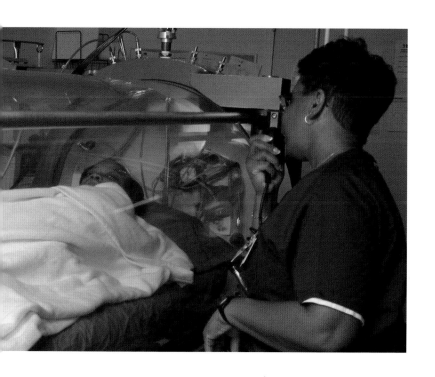

Breakthroughs *in* American Medicine

Tom Nugent

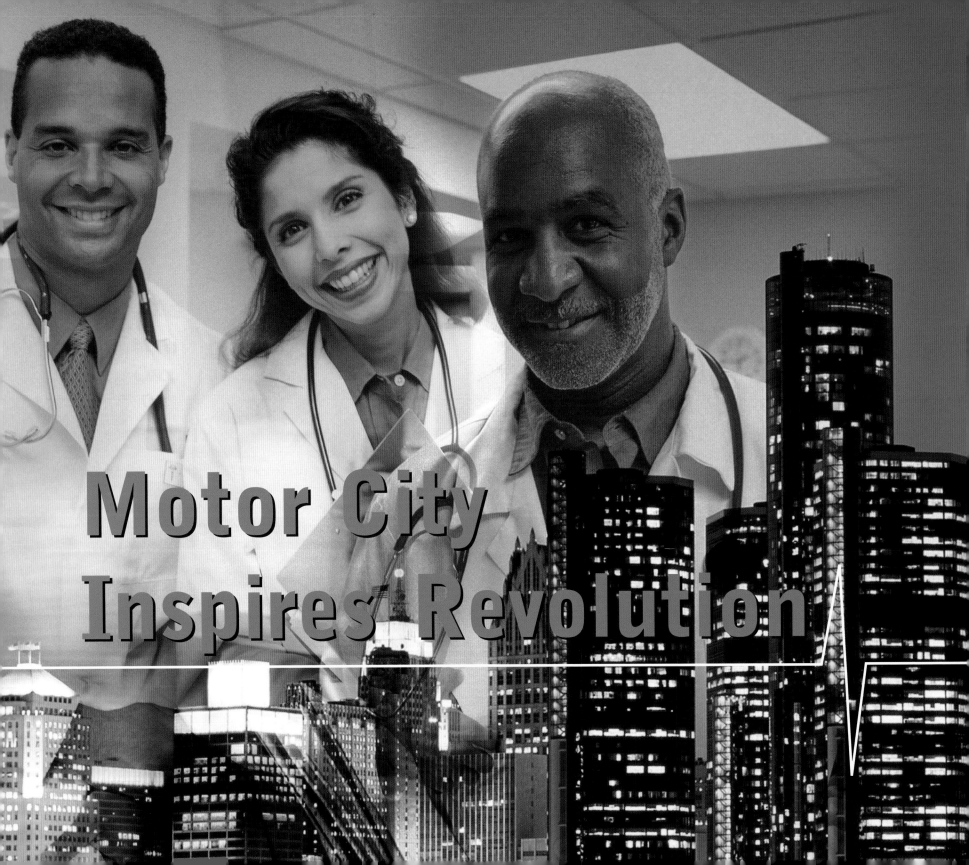

Motor City
Inspires Revolution

"Can-do" spirit inspires health care breakthroughs

They don't call it the "Motor City" for nothing.

During more than a century of global leadership in the manufacture of automobiles, mighty Detroit has fully earned its reputation as the "automotive capital of the world."

But did you know that this 300-year-old metropolis on the Detroit River has also been earning plaudits all across the globe for its innovative breakthroughs in medical treatment and research during recent years?

It's true. And it's a bit surprising to hear, at first. If you're like most Americans, you probably learned in school about the great "auto pioneers" of the early 20th century, legendary figures whose last names (Henry Ford, Ransom Olds, David Buick) speak volumes about the rise of the worldwide auto industry.

If you're like most of us, however, you probably never heard of Dr. Forest Dewey Dodrill, the great Wayne State University and Harper Hospital surgeon who performed the world's first "open-heart" surgery in 1952, right here in Motown.

And how about Lystra E. Gretter, the universally acknowledged health care genius who almost single-handedly created the modern practice of nursing at Harper Hospital in the late 19th century and who, in 1893, wrote the famed "Nightingale Pledge" that is still recited by graduating Registered Nurses throughout the U.S. today?

Pretty impressive, right? But open-heart surgery and science-based nursing are only two of the medical breakthroughs that have put southeast Michigan on the health care map in recent decades. And for good reason. With two of the nation's top 25 medical research universities (Wayne State University and the University of Michigan) located in southeast Michigan — along with leading schools of pharmacy and the country's only National Institutes of Health research campus outside Maryland (in neonatal and premature birth studies) headquartered in midtown Detroit — it's no accident that the "Motor City" is also becoming known as the "Medical City" among health care professionals from Maine to California.

In today's rapidly evolving, information-based economy, the same "can-do" manufacturing culture that made Detroit a world leader in automobiles is providing the creative energy for a similar revolution in medicine and health technology.

Whether we're building a brand-new research center for the National Cancer Institute (southeast Michigan now has two) — or the authoritative neonatal study that promises to help mitigate the effects of PPH by using a pediatric cooling blanket — or conducting the largest study of hypertension among African-Americans in the history of medicine (at Detroit's Receiving Hospital), there's no doubt that the "Motor City" is also becoming the "City of Medical Breakthroughs" at an astonishingly rapid pace.

A thrilling prospect? You bet. And the most exciting part — as you're about to discover in these pages — is that it's already happening, right now and right here in southeast Michigan.

Table of Contents

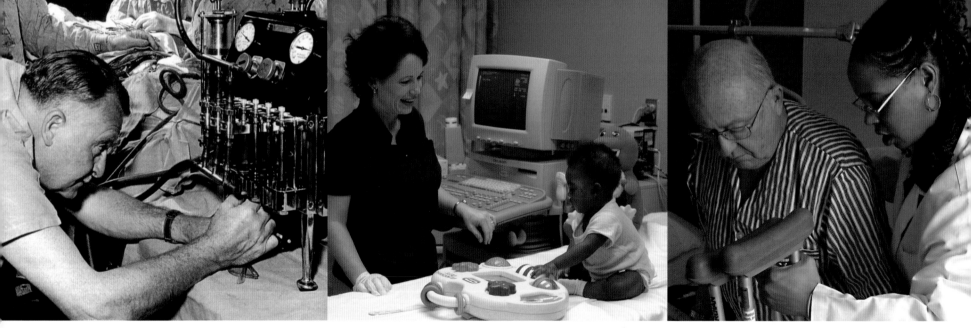

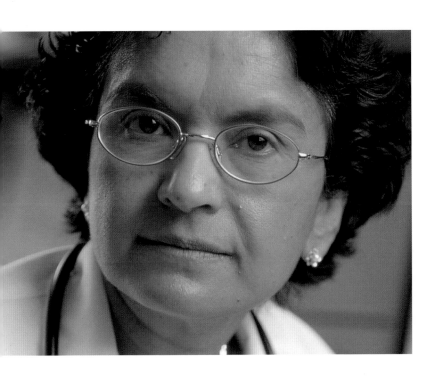

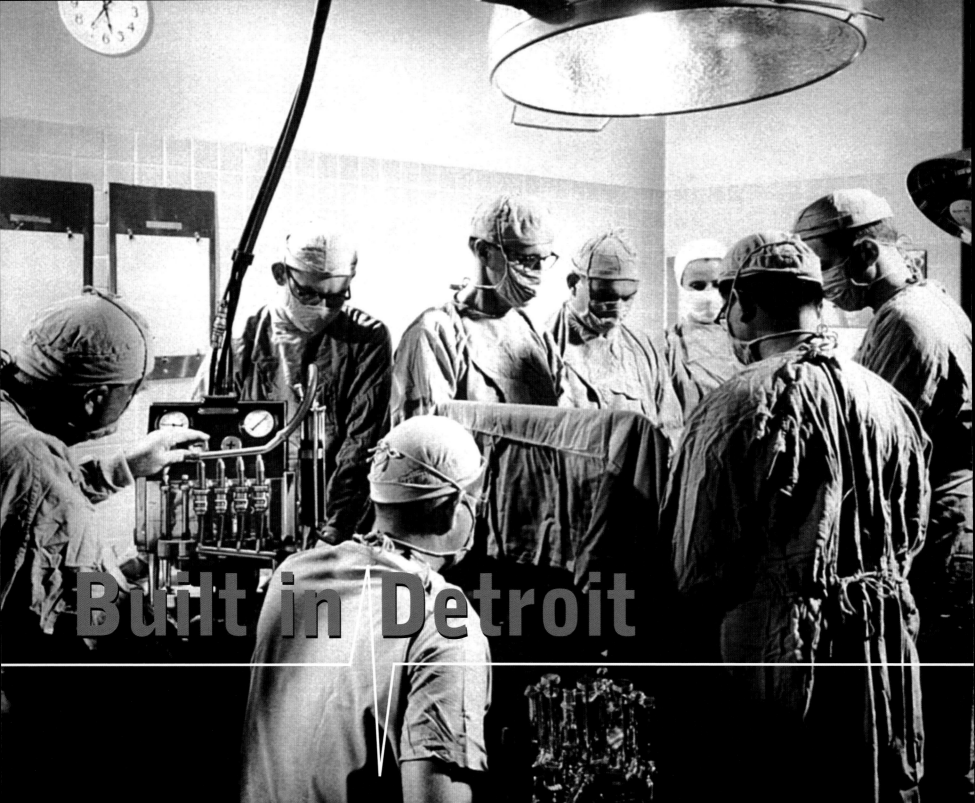

Built in Detroit

Cadillac-like engine pumps away to first successful open-heart surgery

The patient lay motionless on the operating room table. His ailing heart was about to stop beating. The worried surgeons looked at each other for a moment. Then they turned to confront the General Motors engineer who stood beside the strange-looking device plugged directly into the patient's open chest.

With a quick nod, the chief surgeon signaled the GM auto engineer to activate the series of glass pumping chambers that flanked the unconscious, 41-year-old man on the table.

A moment later, the newly invented machine was pumping blood throughout the patient's body and the first successful open-heart surgical procedure in the history of medicine was fully under way.

It happened in a crowded operating room at the Detroit Medical Center's (DMC's) Harper University Hospital on a hot summer morning half a century ago. And it forever changed the way physicians and surgeons go about the critically important task of treating heart disease.

How significant was that dramatic operation for the future of open-heart surgery? Today, this routine procedure is successfully undergone by more than one million patients each year with a risk-of-death factor of less than 1 percent.

"There's no doubt that this was a huge moment in the development of new surgical techniques for heart patients," says Dr. Larry Stephenson, now the chief of cardiac surgery at Harper, the site of the pioneering breakthrough in July 1952.

"What happened in the Harper

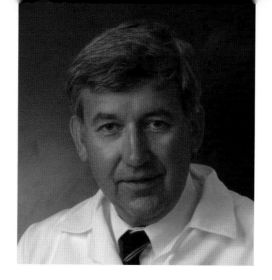

"There's no doubt that this was a huge moment in the development of new surgical techniques for heart patients."

- Larry Stephenson, M.D.

operating room that day had enormous significance for the development of heart-lung machines that have since saved hundreds of thousands of lives all across the globe," Stephenson says.

A veteran cardiac surgeon who has performed more than 6,000 open-heart procedures during his 26-year career, Stephenson credits the surgical team that first used the artificial "Michigan Heart" blood-pumping machine with "displaying an amazing amount of courage in the face of the unknown.

"Let's face it, those guys were confronting some major risks during the operation," says Stephenson the Detroit heart specialist, who recently chronicled the landmark event in a best-selling health book, *State of the Heart* (Write Stuff Enterprises). "For starters, everyone in the operating room knew that if the specially designed GM pump they were using should develop even a small leak in the tubing, air would enter the circuit and then go directly to the patient's brain where it would probably cause a fatal stroke.

"But there were many other hazards as well. I think everyone involved that day knew they were standing on the frontier of heart surgery, and that many of the risks they faced could not have been predicted in advance. And yet they went ahead! Fortunately, their 'Michigan Heart' machine went on to enjoy many years of improved health, and the stage was set for the eventual development of today's remarkably effective heart-lung machines. "I think the story of how they pulled it off still ranks as one of the most thrilling narratives in the history of cardiac surgery."

GM Blood-Pump Resembled "V-12" Cadillac Engine

The world's first successful open-heart operation — performed July 3, 1952 on a Polish-born Detroit resident named Henry Opitek — would make newspaper headlines around the world and for good reason: In the years immediately after World War II, the development and successful deployment of the Michigan Heart provided a vivid example of American know-how and ingenuity in the world of science.

As the DMC's Larry Stephenson is quick to point out, the creation of the first mechanical blood-pump was a joint project that tapped the skills of a gifted Harper Hospital physician along with several Wayne State University medical professors and a team of high-powered engineers from nearby General Motors.

The project kicked off in earnest during the late 1940s when Harper chest surgeon Dr. Forest Dewey Dodrill assembled a high-tech team of medical experts and engineers to create a device that would pump blood throughout the body, thus allowing surgeons to operate directly on the heart for the first time ever.

For the patient, the development of this exciting new tool would be a godsend.

While suffering through a bout of rheumatic fever as a child, Opitek had sustained major damage to a heart valve. Unless he received help soon, the already short-of-breath patient would die from the defect, which obstructed blood flow and allowed blood to be pumped backwards ("regurgitated") from his damaged mitral valve, resulting in a dangerously ineffective heart action.

Dodrill's challenge: Use the new GM-engineered pump to keep blood moving through Opitek's body while the daring physician "turned off" Opitek's heart, then re-opened and strengthened the balky valve with his surgical tools. In the end, the successful repair of the valve would require 14 agonizing minutes, during which the mechanical heart assumed the task of moving the patient's blood through his veins and arteries.

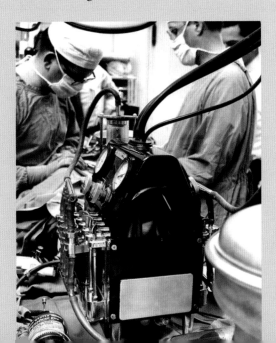

The results were nothing less than spectacular. After spending a few weeks in the hospital, the healthy patient would go on to enjoy more than two decades of an active, energetic life, an outcome that could have been predicted by reading Dr. Dodrill's case report. As the daring surgeon pointed out soon after the operation: "The clinical examination indicates there is a definite improvement. To our knowledge, this is the first instance of survival of a patient when a mechanical heart mechanism was used to take over the complete body function of maintaining the blood supply of the body while the heart was open and operated on."

It took the team of Harper/Wayne State docs and General Motors engineers several years — and half a dozen failed efforts — to build the perfect machine for the job. Describing the immense challenge they faced, GM engineer Ed Rippingille quipped to reporters as the high-profile project got under way, "We've pumped oil, gasoline, water and other fluids in our [automobile] business. It seems only logical we should try to pump blood!"

Another key figure in the development of the Michigan Heart was Charles P. Schaefer, then a "journeyman model maker" in the GM main research lab on Milwaukee Avenue in Detroit. By employing various lengths of stainless steel tubing and a series of glass cylinders, Schaefer was able to translate Rippingille's drawings into an efficient heart pump after nearly two years of full-time effort.

"I made most of the parts for the heart pump myself, and it was quite a job," says Schaefer, the retired technician, now 86 years old. "We were building all kinds of engine parts and other devices in those days. You name it and we could build it!"

Recalls Schaefer, who would spend 36 years working in GM research labs before retiring to Tucson, Arizona in 1983: "In order to build the heart pump, we spent a lot of time developing cam shafts and other components. Mr. Rippingille would design the parts with the help of two other young engineers, Howard Carroll and Lou Self. They showed us what they needed on paper, and then we would build the actual parts to scale.

"For a couple years in the early 1950s, building that pump was pretty much my full-time job," says Schaefer today, "and we were pretty excited about the challenge we faced. We felt a great sense of pride because we knew we were working for the best industrial laboratory in the world."

Schaefer says he vividly recalls the front-page news stories that followed the heart operation on Henry Opitek in July of 1952. "Most of us were really thrilled to be part of that historical moment," he says. "It was very challenging and exciting to work in the GM labs because they usually left us alone to develop our projects, and we had a great deal of engineering freedom."

But Charlie Schaefer's ingenuity wasn't restricted to the Michigan Heart. During the mid-1960s, he and his crew of lab technicians would also design and manufacture several key components for the lunar landing module Eagle, which accomplished the first Apollo landing on the moon in July 1969.

"I worked on the wheels and shafts, and it was a huge job," says Schaefer. "The shafts needed a super-finish, and that required a great deal of teamwork. But we rose to the challenge, and it was our pride in the lab that kept us meeting our deadlines and getting the work out."

Although the expert surgeons at the DMC had great confidence in Charlie Schaefer's heart pump, they also knew that the first human bypass operation posed some unavoidable risks.

"Dodrill showed a great deal of

courage in that operation," says Larry Stephenson, the DMC heart surgeon whose recent history documents the procedure in dramatic detail, "because he and the other members of the team understood full well that if they lost the patient, they would be criticized in many quarters for even having attempted it.

"But the device — which looked remarkably like one of those old 'V-12' Cadillac engines with its 12 glass pumps all working away — worked to perfection," Stephenson adds. They faced very few problems, and finished the procedure sooner than they'd expected.

"Soon publications like *Time Magazine* were referring to the pump as the 'Michigan Heart' in their stories because the Michigan Heart Association [now the Michigan Chapter of the American Heart Association] had also played a major part in putting the huge project together."

Born from the Legacy of Charles Kettering

Like Dr. Stephenson, former General Motors Research Laboratories physicist Bernard Joseph is convinced that the development of the Michigan Heart now ranks as one of the "greatest moments" in the history of 20th century medicine. "I was working in the GM labs on several projects related to optics when the operation took place," Joseph told *Michigan History* magazine in a recent interview, "and I've never forgotten the excitement we felt when the news broke.

"The project had been kept pretty hush-hush until then, but many of us who were working in the labs had heard about it. And when the word came down that the GM pump had saved the patient's life, you could feel a wave of euphoria roll over the entire facility," Joseph remembers. "We were all very proud of the work we were doing in those days in the GM labs, and now the outside world was also recognizing it.

"Most of us just looked at each other and said 'Wow!' Suddenly, the Michigan Heart was in *Time Magazine*, and it was being featured in newspapers all across the country," recalls the 76-year-old Joseph, who retired in 1986. "For those of us working in research at GM, the news meant that the outside world was beginning to recognize the importance of what we were doing in the labs."

According to Joseph, GM's involvement in the project was the direct result of an "enlightened attitude about research" that had been inspired a few years earlier by "the immortal Charles Kettering," the legendary inventor and GM executive who directed research at the auto giant for more than 20 years until his retirement in 1947. His inventions included ethyl gasoline, freon refrigerant and high compression automobile engines

"Kettering had been retired for a few years when I went to work in the labs," Joseph recalls today, "but he was still the 'Emeritus Director,' and he often dropped by to see what we were up to."

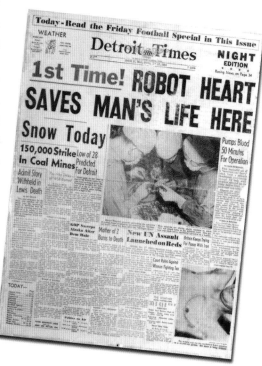

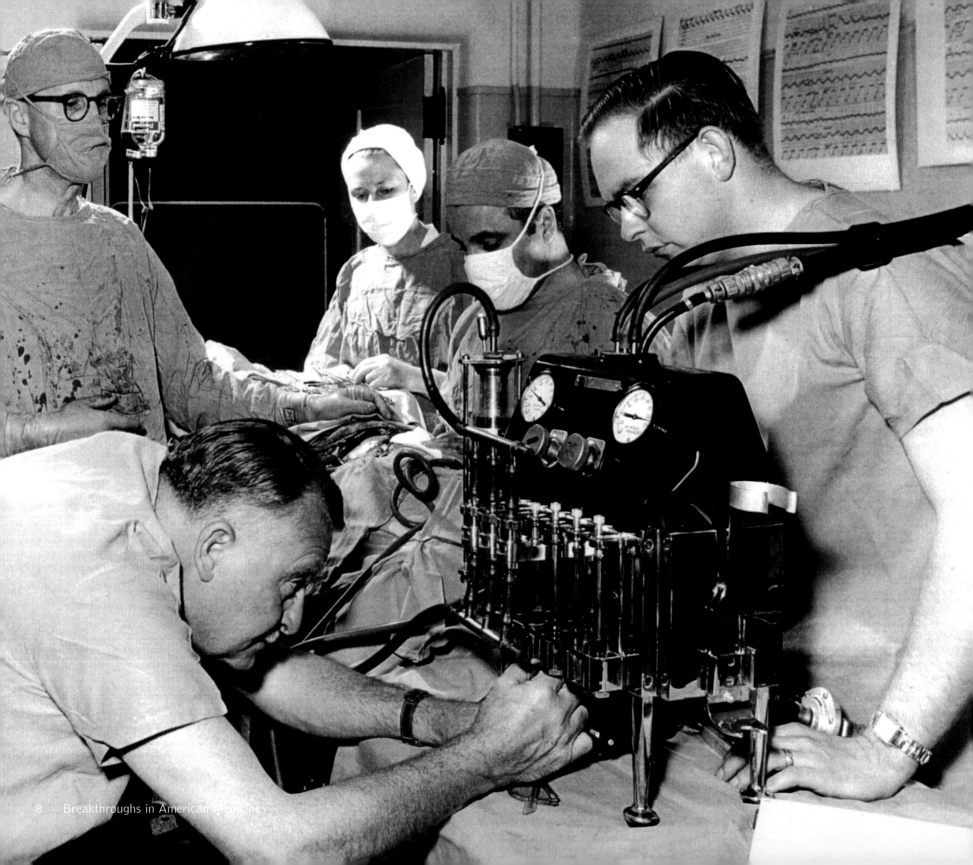

And he was a powerful presence, let me tell you. Kettering was a great big guy, and you'd be standing there working at your lab table, and suddenly you'd feel his presence behind you.

"You would look back over one shoulder, and Kettering would boom at you: 'Hey, young man, what are you doing there? What kind of experiment are you working on?'

"I really think it was because of Charles Kettering — the energy and enthusiasm he brought to those labs throughout his career — that we wound up creating the Michigan Heart. In those days, of course, General Motors was interested in all kinds of different scientific research, and it's no accident that Kettering and Al Sloan [Alfred P. Sloan Jr., GM President from 1923-37] put together one of the world's great cancer research facilities [the Sloan-Kettering Institute, established in 1945]."

Adds the hard-charging Bernard Joseph, a specialist in optics who played a key role in developing the modern automobile headlight now used in more than 90 percent of the world's cars: "I really think the work that went on in the GM labs back in the 1950s and 1960s is one of the 'untold stories' of our time. Most of us took enormous pride in our jobs, and it was a thrilling place to work.

First-ever surgery inspires 25-year-old med student

She remembers the moment when the General Motors engineer threw the switch, remembers the gentle thumping of the pistons — their steady, comforting rhythm — as the world's first mechanical heart began to pump Henry Opitek's blood throughout his unconscious body.

She was a 25-year-old medical student on that July morning in 1952, and she understood that she was witnessing a watershed moment in the history of medicine.

"There were three of us students standing on a raised platform at the back of the operating room," says Dr. Ruth Campbell today. "We wore gowns and sterile caps, and they warned us not to touch *anything*.

"It was a thrilling moment, to say the least. I had been dreaming of becoming a surgeon since I was 10 years old and there I was, watching the first [successful] open-heart surgery ever performed!"

After earning her medical degree a few years later, Ruth Campbell would go on to become the first female surgeon in the history of Harper University Hospital and then to enjoy a 31-year career as a "general surgeon" at the DMC facility.

Now an "emeritus" physician who still works a full day at the DMC's Occupational Health Center, this graceful *eminence* of the DMC surgical world says she has never forgotten her youthful excitement on that long-ago morning in Operating Room No. 12 at Harper.

"We stood on that platform and our eyes were going everywhere," she recalls with a rush of youthful excitement. "Everyone was keyed up about the surgery, but they didn't appear to be rattled.

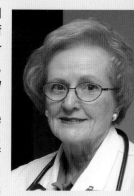

Ruth Campbell, M.D.

"Of course, we all understood that the stakes were very high. If the mechanical heart had failed or if it had developed an air bubble, then there was a distinct possibility that the patient would have died.

"But the surgeons and the residents remained very cool. Dr. [Forest Dewey] Dodrill [the chief surgeon] was quite calm and always such a gentleman. He was a quiet but very authoritative presence in that operating room. Every once in a while, he would turn to Calvin Hughes, the GM research biologist, and the two of them would talk together, but in such low voices that we couldn't hear the words.

"It all seemed to go very smoothly. Mr. Hughes was running the controls on his heart machine, the device was pumping away and Dr. Dodrill was working on the patient. Before we knew it, the operation was over and it seemed clear that the patient would survive."

During the next three decades, as she directed the action in her own Harper operating rooms, General Surgeon Ruth Campbell would often remember the moment when Mr. Hughes threw his switch and ushered in a brand-new era in heart surgery.

"I felt privileged to be there," she says with a quiet smile. "I think I saw the very best of medicine in my day, and watching the first open-heart operation was an unforgettable start to what has been a deeply rewarding career in medicine."

"The Michigan Heart project was a great example of the energy and enthusiasm most of us felt as we worked on our projects, day in and day out," says Joseph.

Another GM retiree who vividly recalls the Michigan Heart project, former, longtime General Motors research engineer Bill Spreitzer, says the dramatic announcement that the Harper-GM team had saved Henry Opitek's life made a "strong impression" on him. "As I learned more about GM's contributions to medical science," remembers Spreitzer, "I realized that I was working for a great company that was determined to provide public services without expectations of recognition or returns.

"We often tend to overlook the many outside contributions made by companies in the industrial world," says Spreitzer, "but the Michigan Heart operation showed the entire world that the work taking place in the labs could be of enormous benefit to the public."

For many observers of the day, the public-spirited nature of the project could be seen clearly in the way the operation was financed. When it came time to pay the medical bills, the delighted Opitek discovered that the physicians involved had all donated their services and that his entire hospital charge after a stay of several weeks at the miniscule sum of only $14 per night had amounted to only $340!

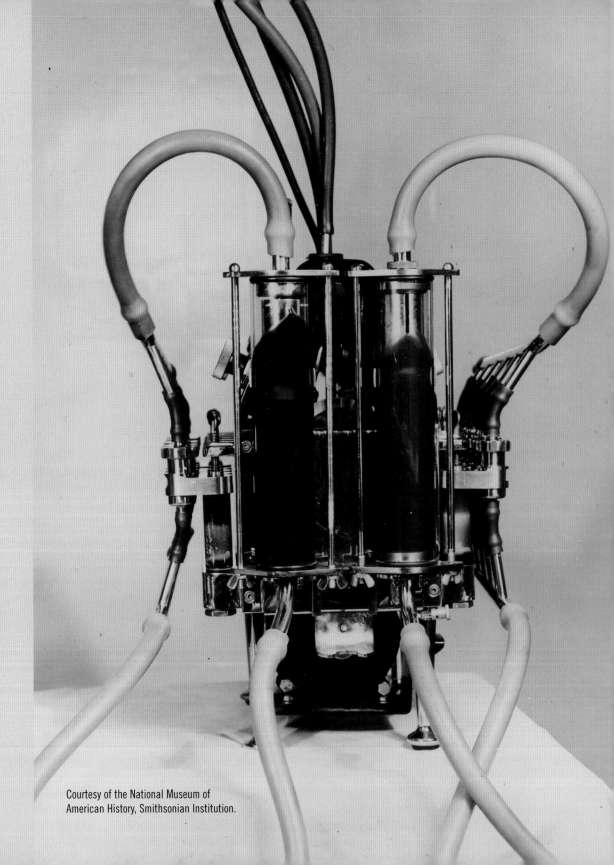

Courtesy of the National Museum of American History, Smithsonian Institution.

Still on Display
at the Smithsonian

Only a few months after the successful operation on Henry Opitek, the story of the Michigan Heart took another amazing twist when several skilled machinists from GM's auto research lab were asked to help Dodrill & Co. build a smaller model of the pump for a young child with a dangerous heart defect.

The machinists were happy to oblige, but they also happened to be walking a United Auto Workers (UAW) picket line at that time as part of an ongoing labor strike against GM.

The solution? At the urging of the automaker, UAW officials quickly agreed to allow the machinists to cross their picket line. They did the job in a flash, and the young girl's life was saved in the operation that soon followed. To honor the technological breakthrough, the Smithsonian Institution put the Michigan Heart on permanent display in Washington, D.C., where it remains to this day. (Other versions of the famous pump can also be found on display at the GM Heritage Center and in the lobby of Harper University Hospital.)

Ask Larry Stephenson to describe the bottom-line significance of that long-ago day in the operating room at Harper Hospital, and the veteran heart surgeon doesn't miss a beat. "It's amazing when you realize that only 50 years ago, a patient with even a simple heart defect was just plain out of luck. That person was doomed to an early death whether the problem was a birth defect or a blockage in a coronary artery.

"But these days, virtually all of those heart problems can be corrected with open-heart surgery, and the risk is only about one percent for many procedures. Think of it: 99 of those 100 people will live today thanks to the new techniques and the heart-lung machines that have evolved from the Michigan Heart."

"It's amazing when you realize that only 50 years ago, a patient with even a simple heart defect was just plain out of luck."

- Larry Stephenson, M.D.

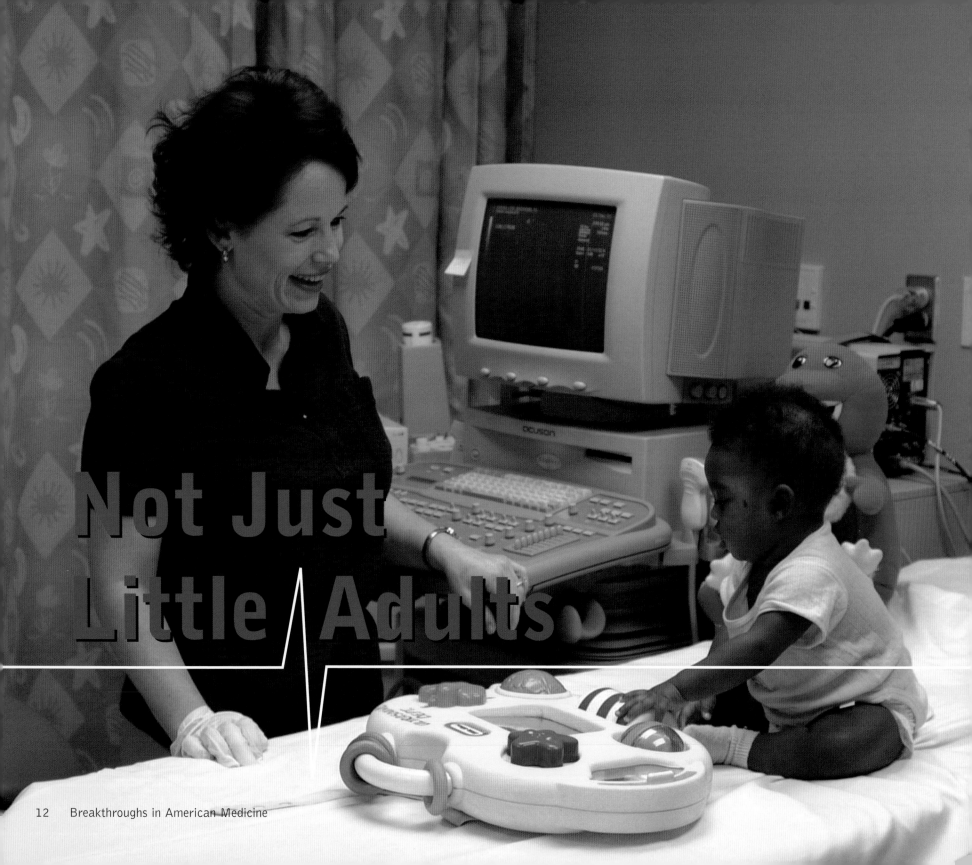

Not Just
Little Adults

An advocate for better health care for kids

Take a brief stroll through the busy surgical suites at Children's Hospital of Michigan, where 30 full-time surgeons perform more than 12,000 operations on kids each year, and it's easy to assume that the medical specialty known as "pediatric surgery" was always a thriving enterprise.

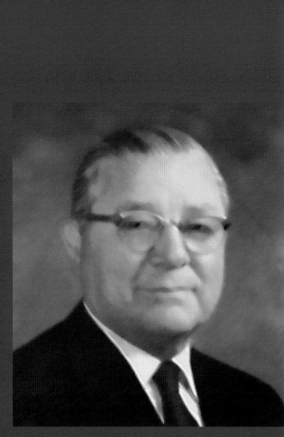

Clifford D. Benson, M.D.
Winner of the prestigious William E. Ladd Medal from the American Academy of Pediatrics for his significant contribution to the field of pediatric surgery in 1982.

Not true, says veteran DMC physician Michael Klein.

"Believe it or not, the doctors who created and developed pediatric surgery in the 1950s and 1960s had to fight very hard in order to get their specialty recognized," says Dr. Klein, the chief of pediatric surgery at CHM since 1991. "There was tremendous opposition to the idea that surgeons should specialize in treating children. Children were often regarded by physicians as simply being 'little adults,' and many surgeons assumed they could operate without the need for any special preparation."

But all of that has changed in recent years, says the high-octane DMC doc. That's thanks in part to the courageous leadership shown by a former Children's pediatric surgeon, Dr. Clifford D. Benson, who became a nationally renowned figure in the struggle to establish the field as an accepted medical specialty.

Frequently described by former U.S. Surgeon General C. Everett Koop (also a pediatric surgeon) as a "beloved colleague" who helped put pediatric surgery on the map, the legendary Dr. Benson spent several decades performing surgery on Detroit-area kids, even as he assembled and then managed a high-profile surgical team at Children's in the 1960s and 1970s.

"Cliff Benson was a real hero, a true pioneer in his field," says Dr. Klein today. "During the 1960s, he built one of the nation's best pediatric surgery departments right here at Children's. He was a widely admired surgeon, and he edited one of the first textbooks on pediatric surgery.

"But his biggest contribution, it seems to me, was the unflagging leadership he showed in getting pediatric surgery recognized as a unique and autonomous field of medicine. And that took a great deal of courage, believe me, because there was some powerful resistance from such entrenched groups as the American College of Surgeons and the American Board of Surgery."

Like Dr. Klein, Children's Hospital of Michigan President Dr. Larry E. Fleischmann says he has long been "a great admirer of Cliff Benson and the major role he played nationally in supporting the development of pediatric surgery.

"There's no doubt that the early pioneers faced an uphill struggle," says the longtime pediatric nephrology specialist, who took the helm at Children's

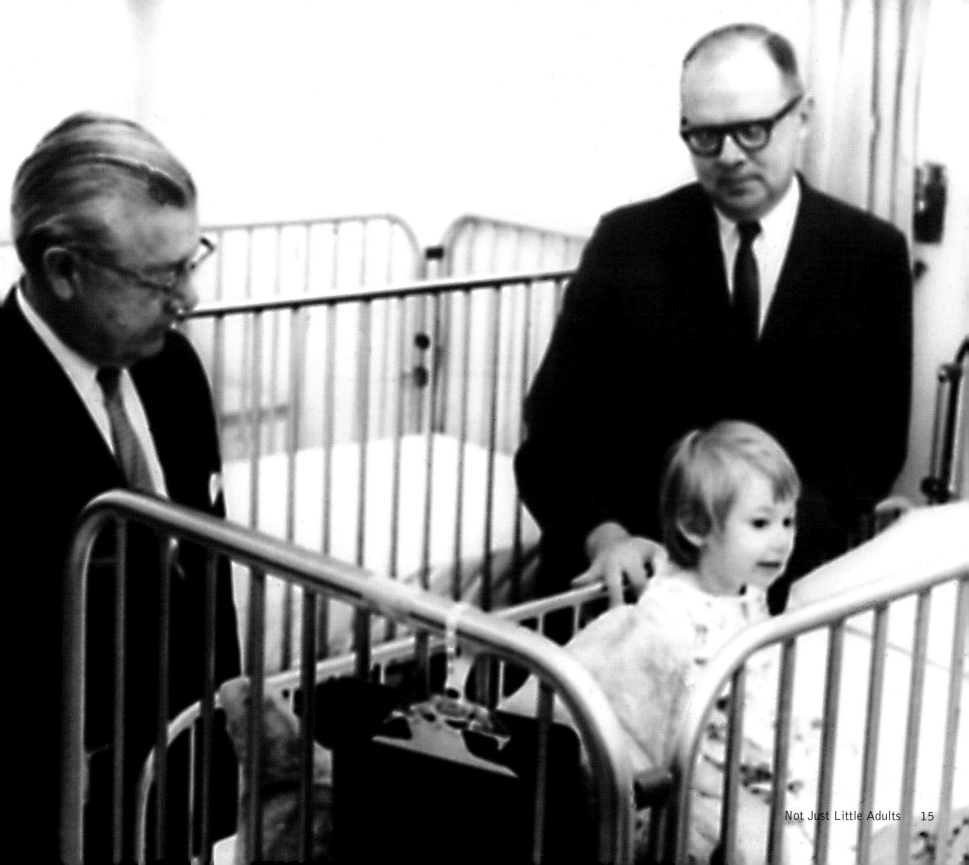

in 1998 and who was preparing for retirement in the summer of 2005. "When the idea of having surgical specialists for children came in, a lot of general surgeons were opposed. And they would tell you, 'I can do that [pediatric surgery] as well as anybody, and there's no need for a specialist.'

"But that statement simply wasn't true," says Dr. Fleischmann, a noted kidney expert who founded the CHM's highly regarded Renal Dialysis and Treatment program after joining the hospital staff in 1968. "These days, most physicians understand that the more you study a particular area of surgery, the better you will know it, and the better able you will be to practice it."

Dr. Benson, won the prestigious William E. Ladd Medal from the American Academy of Pediatrics for his significant contribution to the field of pediatric surgery in 1982. He displayed a passionate commitment to the health and welfare of children throughout his long career at the CHM, according to Dr. Klein.

"Practicing pediatrics in the 1950s and early 1960s was very difficult at times," he explains, "because Medicaid hadn't been created yet, and the pay rate for doctors who treated kids was quite low. As a result, many of the first

The Jackie Robinson of kids surgery

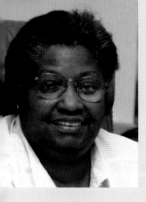

Alexa Canady, M.D.

They call her "the Jackie Robinson of pediatric neurosurgery." Her two decades as chief of neurosurgery were key in building a national reputation for excellence at the DMC's major medical facility for kids.

"There's no doubt that Alexa Canady was a pioneer in her field," says Dr. Larry Fleishmann. Until retirement [in 2001], she directed groundbreaking surgery that became a model for similar programs across the country. Dr. Canady was a compassionate doctor with a fierce determination to treat children struggling with the most severe neurologic disorders.

She routinely worked a 14-hour day while also finding time to conduct research and publish it in some of the nation's leading scientific journals.

As the youngest African-American neurosurgeon to practice in the U.S., the indefatigable Dr. Canady was often compared to the great major league baseball player Jackie Robinson, who broke through the "color barrier" in pro baseball. But Dr. Canady wasn't particularly interested in celebrating that

aspect of her astonishing career; most of her energy went into treating sick kids and the struggle to win acceptance for pediatric neurosurgery as an autonomous medical specialty in American medicine.

Dr. Canady's personal story — as a young, black physician from Lansing, Michigan who refused to be intimidated by her "minority status" in medical school at the University of Michigan and during later surgical residencies at hospitals in Connecticut, Minnesota and Pennsylvania — was much larger than a mere story of a woman "succeeding against the odds." She also served as a powerful source of inspiration for women and African-Americans across a wide spectrum of professional life.

"I loved working at Children's," she says today. "It was joyous! It gave me a marvelous opportunity to work with people who were trying to do the right thing. That attitude permeated everything we did, and we were all immensely proud of the fact that every child who came to our hospital received treatment, regardless of ability to pay.

"It was hard work at times, and we did put in some long days. But the journey was certainly worth the effort."

pediatricians faced significant financial hardship, including Cliff Benson. I've heard that he wound up getting in some real financial trouble toward the end of his life, and it happened because he'd spent so many years treating children for free."

Dr. Klein is also careful to point out that "the battle to help children with surgery and other treatments is far from over. I do think the word 'fight' is the correct word to use in describing how many pediatricians feel about their role as advocates for better children's medical care," he will tell you with a lighthearted chuckle.

"I believe most of us choose to be pediatric surgeons because we're drawn to kids. And that was certainly the case with Cliff Benson. He was a terrific clinician, of course, and also a technological innovator who developed and refined a key surgical procedure for infants born with pyloric stenosis [a congenital defect that causes harmful narrowing of the upper stomach].

"Dr. Benson was a skilled physician," Dr. Klein recalls, "but everyone who knew him recognized that he was also a terrific advocate for better health care for kids."

Trained as a physician at Case Western Reserve University in Cleveland, the affable Dr. Klein says he shares Dr. Benson's passion for treating children with surgery at Children's Hospital of Michigan. He's also pleased by the fact that his 120-year-old pediatric hospital now treats more than 60,000 children each year.

"Kids are wonderful!" he announces with a boom of sudden laughter when you ask him to explain why he chose a career in pediatrics.

Then, in an aside that echoes most of the other 29 pediatric surgeons on call daily at the CHM: "The great thing about having children for patients is that they're usually very nice people — and sometimes you even get to hug 'em!"

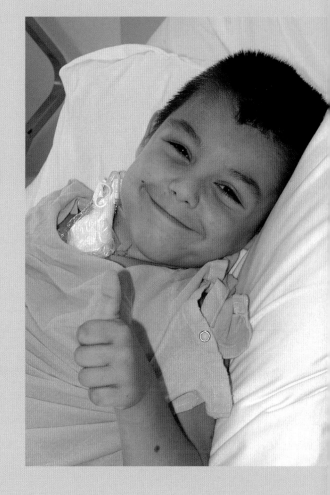

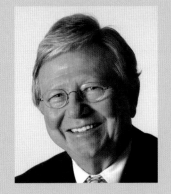

"These days, most physicians understand that the more you study a particular area of surgery, the better you will know it, and the better able you will be to practice it."

- Larry E. Fleischmann, M.D.

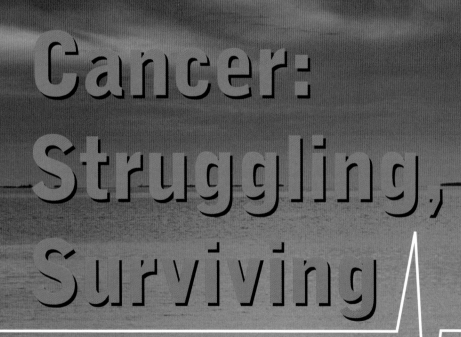

Cancer: Struggling, Surviving

Struggling patient won victory against a deadly tumor

Every once in awhile, Dr. Donald W. Weaver gets another grateful postcard from his pal in Muskegon. The Muskegon pal — let's call him "Charlie" — is a former cancer patient at the Detroit Medical Center.

About 10 years ago, Charlie visited Donald W. Weaver, M.D., in his consulting rooms at Harper University Hospital. Dr. Weaver is Professor and Chairman of the Department of Surgery, Wayne State University School of Medicine and Surgeon-in-Chief of the Detroit Medical Center. Looking downcast and depressed, the patient told the veteran Detroit cancer surgeon a grim story that seemed certain to end in tragedy.

"Unfortunately, this patient was struggling with a large tumor in his liver and he'd already been told by several physicians that it would be impossible to remove it," recalls Dr. Weaver today. "At that point, he was pretty much out of options, and he'd begun to wonder if his life might be approaching its end.

"But the good news for this patient was that the surgical staff at the DMC has been specializing in tumors of the liver and pancreas in recent years. By using the very latest surgical techniques and recently devised tools such as radio-frequency and cryogenic ablation in conjuction with state-of-the-art resection techniques, we have been able to address these difficult-to-manage liver tumors with a surprising degree of success."

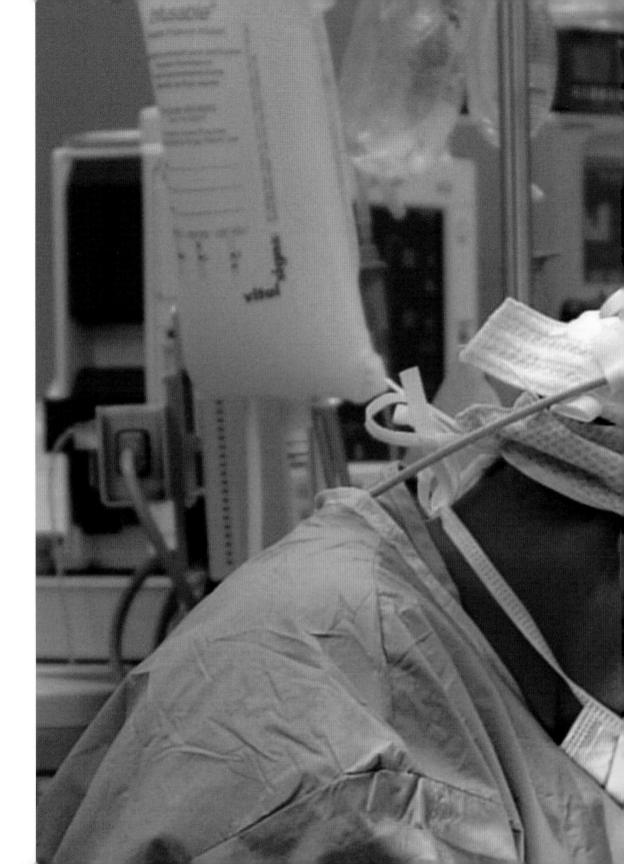

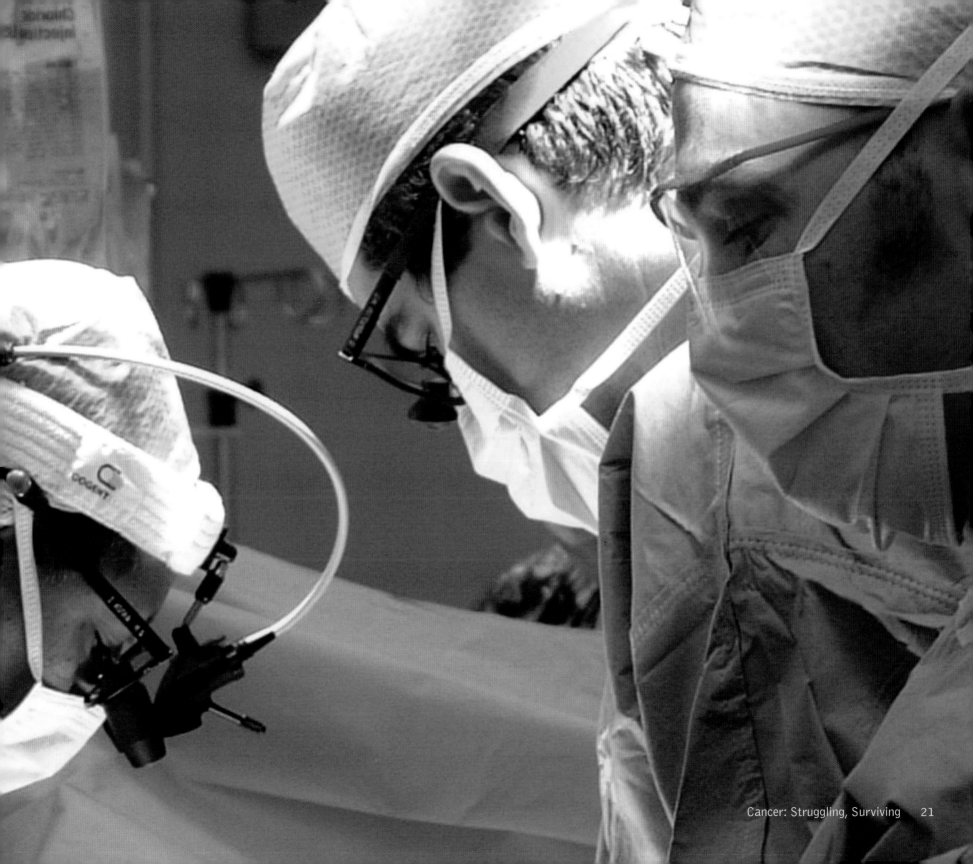

After examining Charlie carefully and studying his medical history in great detail, Dr. Weaver and his team of DMC surgeons surprised the patient by challenging the assumption that his liver cancer was inoperable.

"Operating on the liver and on the pancreas — these are probably the two most complex and difficult kinds of cancer surgery in medicine today," says the 55-year-old Dr. Weaver, who has spent the past 25 years as a surgeon at the DMC. "Still, these kinds of tumors *can* be addressed with surgery under the right conditions. In this particular case, we told the patient that we thought it would be possible to operate successfully on his liver tumor. We warned him that the road ahead would surely be difficult, but we also held out the hope for a positive outcome."

What followed, says Dr. Weaver, was a long, hard climb up a very steep hill.

"Over the years, I've come to think of cancer surgery as being a little bit like mountain-climbing," he will tell you with a quiet smile. "And I sometimes will tell a patient, 'If you're going to try to climb Mt. Everest, you'll need a professional mountain guide to walk every step of the way with you.'"

In this case, the patient listened carefully and then decided to proceed. With ongoing advice and daily encouragement, the struggling Charlie underwent a complex surgical procedure for his liver cancer under the direction of Dr. Weaver.

"For me, performing cancer surgery on a human being is always a humbling experience. Putting your hands inside somebody's body in an effort to help them solve a medical issue that's just a

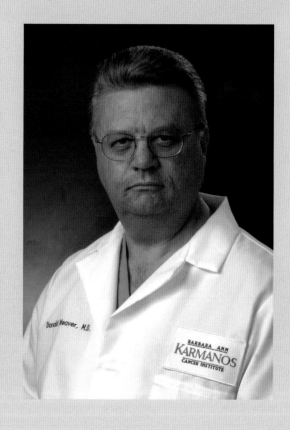

"Operating on the liver and on the pancreas — these are probably the two most complex and difficult kinds of cancer surgery in medicine today."

- Donald W. Weaver, M.D.

very humbling, a very profound kind of event for any doctor.

"I think the key to effective surgery is, above all, good *planning* — careful, detailed planning in which you analyze every single aspect of the procedure again and again while also doing your best to put together an advance plan for dealing with every possible contingency during the operation.

"When cancer surgery goes well and the patient benefits as a result, well, that's a wonderfully encouraging outcome. And if things don't go so well, that's just awful for the surgeon, believe me. That's really terrible for the doctor, and it's always very, very difficult to accept.

"Fortunately, in the case of the gentleman from Muskegon, the outcome was very positive, and all of us were quite pleased by the long-term results."

And what were those "results," exactly?

That question takes us back to the postcard from "Charlie," a card that arrived in Dr. Weaver's office at the DMC in the summer of 2005.

The cheerful postcard noted that Charlie was in the middle of a sailing vacation along Lake Michigan where he was "having a blast" piloting his 27-foot sloop past giant sand dunes and candy-striped lighthouses each day.

As usual, the card then went on to thank Dr. Weaver and his staff for helping the patient to enjoy more than a decade of active, exuberant life after having been diagnosed with an "inoperable" liver cancer that appeared to be terminal.

Describing the recent postcard from his friend of more than a decade, Dr. Weaver lights up with the quiet

joyfulness that forms a key element in his approach to cancer surgery, day in and day out.

"When you read a card like that, when a patient tells you that he's sailing along in his boat and thinking about you and your colleagues with a lot of gratitude, well, that's the kind of message that just makes your entire day."

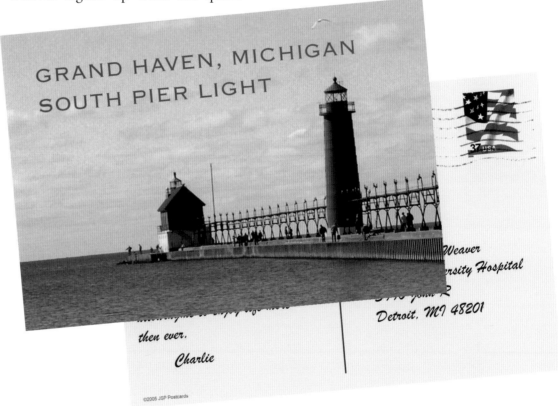

GRAND HAVEN, MICHIGAN
SOUTH PIER LIGHT

then ever.

Charlie

©2005 JSP Postcards

Weaver
...rsity Hospital
Detroit, MI 48201

Cancer survivor sensitive to struggles of young patients

He's a high-profile cancer researcher, a pioneering scientist who made headlines in February of 2005 when his breakthrough co-discovery regarding the treatment of children with acute myeloid leukemia (which typically responds poorly to treatment) was published in the *Journal of the National Cancer Institute.*

Why is Dr. Jeffrey W. Taub, a compassionate veteran oncologist at the DMC Children's Hospital of Michigan, so keenly sensitive to the struggles of his young patients?

It's simple.

When Dr. Taub (now 42) was 14 years old, he learned that he had Hodgkin's disease, a rare type of lymphoma that invades the body's lymphatic system and that often attacks children and teenagers.

But with the help of an outstanding medical team and lots of determination, Jeff Taub survived his disease and went on to become a specialist in pediatric cancer.

In 1996, the story of Dr. Taub's remarkable odyssey took another amazing turn. That's when he met 13-year-old Michelle D. Bailey, a Detroit teenager diagnosed as suffering from Hodgkin's.

During the next year or so, he helped her struggle through an intense regimen of chemotherapy, a strategic deployment of state-of-the-art medications aimed at shutting down the proliferating cancer cells.

Nine years after winning that battle, a healthy Michelle D. Bailey studies diligently at Oakland University en route to what she promises will be a high-voltage teaching career.

Ask Michelle to reflect on her unusual story and she doesn't hesitate: "Dr. Taub had cancer like me, and we were the same age when we got it. When I heard his story, it was so inspirational! He survived and went on to be a doctor who helps kids. I'm so glad I ended up at Children's Hospital because my doctor turned out to be a friend who understood exactly what I was going through."

And Dr. Taub? Ask him to talk about Michelle D. Bailey, and you can hear the affection he feels for her in every word. "That's the really gratifying part of my job," he says quietly, "when they come back for follow-ups, and you can see how well they're doing. When you treat a patient like Michelle, and you see how determined she is to do something useful with her life. That's a huge payback!"

Dr. Taub is a clinician who loves to talk about his patients. But he's equally dedicated to his laboratory research. And that's why he was so pleased in February 2005 when the news broke about his research team's chemotherapy breakthrough in the treatment of a type of leukemia that often attacks youngsters with Down syndrome.

Dr. Taub and fellow researchers discovered that most Down syndrome children can be treated with lower levels of the anti-cancer drug (cytosine arabinoside) than had previously been thought.

Funded by the National Cancer Institute, Dr. Taub's three-year tissue-based study proved conclusively that the leukemia cells in many kids with Down syndrome are far more sensitive to this powerful drug than anyone had thought.

A pediatric cancer specialist since 1991, Dr. Taub says he's deeply committed to both laboratory research and daily clinical treatment of patients at Children's Hospital of Michigan. Why? Because both activities are "absolutely essential" to helping patients like Michelle D. Bailey.

"One of the key motivations for our research at Children's Hospital of Michigan is that we want to keep reducing the side effects of chemotherapy because fewer side effects mean a better quality of life for both the patients and their families. We're looking for better use of medications, better technology solutions, better treatment protocols every time we walk into that lab.

"But we're also doing our best, in clinical terms, to reach out to each and every one of our patients. In Michelle's case, it seemed appropriate to tell her my own story about surviving Hodgkin's. Having lived through that struggle myself, I was determined to stand beside her every step of the way!"

Dr. Taub is The Ring Screw Textron Chair for Pediatric Cancer Research, appointed by the Wayne State University Board of Governors.

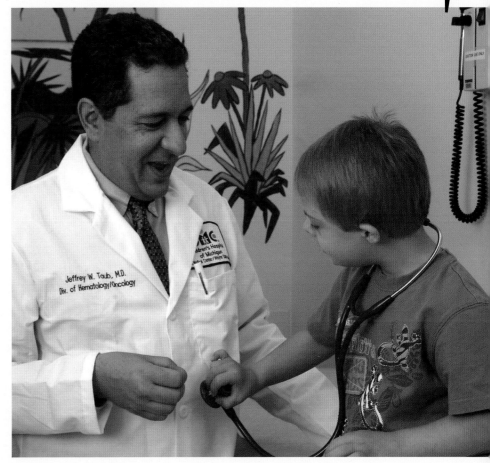

Jefferey W. Taub, M.D.

Taking the Nightingale Pledge

Innovative 1883 program
became model nurse-training
throughout the world

She remembers a mild spring evening back in 1967, remembers standing on a brilliantly lit auditorium stage at Harper University Hospital with tears in her eyes and a lump in her throat.

I SOLEMNLY PLEDGE myself before God and in the presence of this assembly, to pass my life in purity and to practice my profession faithfully. I WILL abstain from whatever is deleterious and mischievous, and will not take or knowingly administer any harmful drug. I WILL do all in my power to maintain and elevate the standard of my profession, and will hold in confidence all personal matters committed to my keeping and all family affairs coming to my knowledge in the practice of my calling. With loyalty will I aid the physician in his work, and as a "missioner of health" I WILL dedicate myself to devoted service to human welfare.

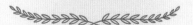

Presented by Hospital Division, Parke, Davis & Company
Copyright 1936, Alumnae Association, Harper Hospital School of Nursing

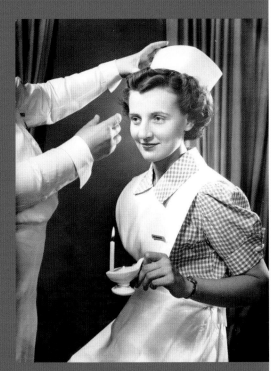

Capping a nursing graduate in 1958.

Nancy Louise Wrublewski — an energetic and very determined young woman from the Polish-American enclave of Hamtramck in the great American city of Detroit — was about to become a Registered Nurse.

She remembers how she raised her right hand, and then joined 50 other graduates in reciting a pledge that had been written more than 70 years before by the distinguished Lystra E. Gretter, who had almost single-handedly created what many observers of the day regarded as one of the world's first modern nursing schools.

The Farrand Training School for Nurses, established at Harper University Hospital in 1883, had been one of the first such institutions in the United States to design and then introduce a disciplined, science-based curriculum aimed at preparing young women for professional careers in nursing.

Led by the formidable, no-nonsense Mrs. Gretter, the Harper University Hospital nursing school had then graduated its first class (four Registered Nurses) in 1885.

By 1890, the ranks of Harper's nurses-in-training would have expanded to more than 60 as the increasingly visible program began attracting more and more candidates from across Michigan and the Midwest.

During the next 77 years, Mrs. Gretter's pioneering program would grow steadily, eventually becoming one of the nation's most highly regarded training rounds for men and women who hoped to win the coveted designation: "R.N."

Flash forward to 1967. . . Nancy Wrublewski raises her right hand and speaks the words of the "Florence Nightingale Pledge," composed by Lystra Gretter at Harper in 1893, and today recited by tens of thousands of brand-new Registered Nurses each year.

Repeating the famous phrases, Wrublewski feels "a powerful connection to the generations of Harper nurses" who have preceded her on this stage:

"I solemnly pledge myself before God and in the presence of this assembly, to pass my life in purity and to practice my profession faithfully. . . . "

Looking back from a distance of nearly four decades, Wrublewski will tell you that studying nursing at Harper Hospital in the mid-1960s was one of the "greatest experiences" of her life.

"That was another world," she will add, with a smile of cheerful nostalgia. And then she'll hold up a pale-gray, checker-cloth nursing uniform, neatly pressed and swaying gently from its hanger. "This is the uniform I wore in school for three years and then later out on the wards at Harper Hospital.

"These nursing uniforms were manufactured in Scotland, we were told, and they went out to nursing schools, hospitals and clinics all across the world. We wore a little muslin cap as well. And when you had completed a year of school, you were allowed to put a stripe on the front of the uniform blouse. That way, we could all tell at a glance how far along we were in the Harper program."

Describing other aspects of the three-year program of studies, she glows with the warmth of vivid memories: "In those days, nursing school was entirely different than it is today. And as students, we all lived very regimented, very controlled lives. Each nurse was assigned a room right in the hospital, for example, and our meals were all eaten in the hospital cafeteria.

"We sent our uniforms — the Scottish ginghams — to the main hospital laundry, and we even had maids who would come around once a week to neaten up our rooms.

"In that world, little things counted for a lot, things like the 'Night Cafeteria,' a delightful little nook where they served hot meals for the hospital staff all night long. Can you imagine? The Night Cafeteria is long gone, of course. Today, a nurse or a doctor would have to rely on vending machines, and it's just not the same."

Another pleasing aspect of 1960s nursing school was the extremely low cost. She recalls that the tuition was only $600 for the entire program and that candidates had to pass a "Standardized Test" in order to be accepted. "I was very fortunate," she recalls today, "because the state of Michigan paid my tuition entirely. I'd been ill for some time before attending nursing school, and the state had a program that allowed candidates in my condition to be exonerated from payments. The state paid the entire cost because Michigan officials were deeply concerned about the chronic shortage of trained nurses.

"I thought that was a great deal, and I felt very privileged to be able to attend three years of nursing school for free!"

While spending several years on the wards at Harper after graduation, Nancy Wrublewski would continue to study nursing at night. In 1972, she would

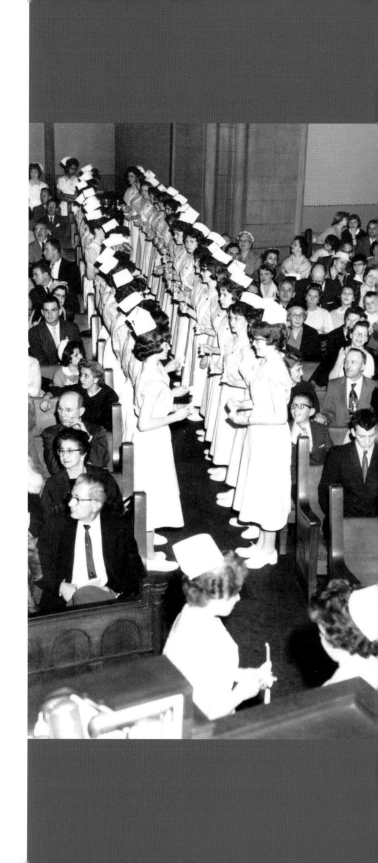

receive a diploma from Wayne State University, and then go on to spend many years as a practicing nurse anesthetist in the Detroit area.

"Thanks to Harper Hospital and the state of Michigan, I was able to enjoy a wonderful career as a nurse," she said recently, a few years after settling into contented retirement.

"Those three years in school at Harper were extremely challenging. We worked hard and we struggled daily to get it right and to become the best nurses we were capable of being. That was a very intense time, a very thrilling time, and I wouldn't have traded it for anything."

Along with Nancy Wrublewski, more than 5,000 Registered Nurses have graduated from the Harper Hospital nursing education program during the more than 120 years since its founding in 1883.

As several medical historians have noted in recent years, the idea of training young women to meet professional nursing standards was actually a brand-new concept during the 1880s. But when an innovative physician at Harper Hospital (Dr. Jacob S. Farrand, the hospital president from 1884-91) learned about the benefits to be gained by schooling nurses in the art and science of medicine, he decided that his hospital should become one of the leading nurse-training facilities in the entire country.

Only a few years before Dr. Farrand's initiative, of course, legendary British nurse Florence Nightingale (1820-1910) had gained fame during the Crimean War by launching professional training programs in nursing throughout the British Empire. During the late 1870s and 1880s, her revolutionary teaching model would be copied by a few American medical centers, which meant that Dr. Farrand in 1883 would be bringing Harper Hospital into the movement right on the ground floor.

Under the Detroit doctor's leadership, the first Harper nursing students were assigned rooms on the hospital's fourth floor from which they could move freely about the facility in order to attend "didactic lectures" and also to assist patients (according to later historians Frank B. Woodford and Philip P. Mason), in " . . . dressing wounds, apply-ing blisters, cups, and leeches, using the catheter, administering enemas, applying friction, bandaging, making beds, changing draw sheets, moving patients, and preventing bedsores."

Within a few years, the Farrand Training School for Nurses at Harper Hospital had begun to win plaudits from physicians and hospital administrators all across the country. As a Harper Hospital committee noted in a special report on the facility in 1886: "The school is now thoroughly organized and first class in all its equipment. The amount of instruction is greater and in many important respects the school is in advance of any similar school in the country."

Only a year later, another Harper committee would praise the new nursing school to the skies while proudly noting: "The School is doing splendid work, and stands so well in public esteem that, out of ninety-four graduates in active service, thirty are now at the head or in responsible positions in other training

"I thought that was a great deal, and I felt very privileged to be able to attend three years of nursing school for free!"

- Nancy Louise Wrublewski

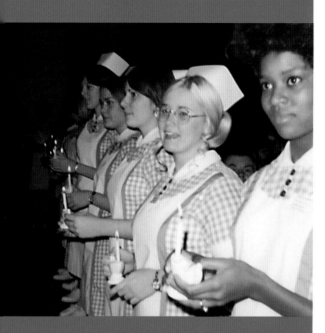

"We have a long and proud history of staffing and helping to develop excellent nurses over several generations."

- Iris A. Taylor, Ph.D., R.N.

schools and hospitals in the United States. This is a record of which the School may well be proud."

Summer, 1917: Treating the Wounded from Battlefields All across France

When the call went out to the American medical community for help on the battlefields of France, the medical professionals from Harper Hospital would respond quickly. With 21 physicians and more than 50 nurses in tow, the Harper contingent in the summer of 1917 would establish "Base Hospital 17," the largest American military hospital to operate in France at the height of World War I.

Established at Dijon, Hospital 17 included 2,000 beds and treated thousands of American and French soldiers alike. Soon the facility would be flooded with wounded soldiers from the great battles that were being fought at Chateau-Thierry, at the Argonne and at St. Mihiel. Here's how Harper historians Woodford and Mason described the Harper contribution to the American war effort:

"For the Harper personnel, Dijon was a far cry from the red brick hospital building on John R Street in Detroit. The unit took over a French hospital housed in an ancient chateau-like structure, which once had been a boys' school. It was a four-story, L-shaped building that had been equipped by the citizens of Dijon using their own spare household articles. It had a bed capacity of only 75, which was soon expanded to 1,800 by the addition of 14 wooden barracks.

"Base Hospital 17 was the first American unit in Dijon except for a detachment of bakers, and the burghers took the Yanks to their hearts."

No sooner had the Armistice been signed, however, than the Harper professionals found themselves neck-deep in yet another health care crisis with the outbreak of the deadly flu epidemic of 1918. In the end, the medical team from Detroit would spend the best part of that year doing their best to treat the tens of thousands of soldiers who came down with the disease.

"Excellent nursing" key to the best medical care

Ask Dr. Iris A. Taylor, President of Detroit Receiving Hospital, to reflect on "the art and science of nursing," and this veteran DMC administrator won't hesitate. "I think you need two things to be a really effective nurse," she says thoughtfully.

"First, you need the ability to assess the needs of the patient and to translate the patient's medical data into a plan that will successfully attain the medical goals established by his or her physicians.

"Second, you need compassion for the human being you're treating. But the essence of good nursing isn't just being 'warm and fuzzy.' Clearly, the essence is to make sure all the clinical needs, psychological needs and social needs of that patient are being met."

During nearly three decades of outstanding service at both the DMC's Receiving Hospital and the University Health Center, Dr. Taylor mastered her nursing skills the old-fashioned way, by working on busy hospital wards as an R.N. and later as a head nurse and vice president of nursing.

After a brief stint in the late 1990s as President and CEO of The Detroit Institute of Children, Dr. Taylor resumed her

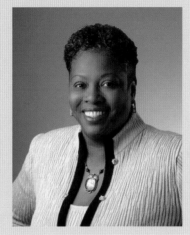

Iris A. Taylor, Ph.D., R.N.

DMC career by signing on in 1999 as Chief Nursing Officer and Senior Vice President of Patient Care. In 2004, she was tapped by the DMC Board of Directors to be President at Receiving.

Describing her vision for the 97-year-old medical facility, Dr. Taylor talks excitedly about what she sees as "a marvelous opportunity to help this hospital develop a whole new line of excellent specialties in such areas as neurology, gerontology and hypertension.

"I don't think there's any doubt that Receiving's biggest claim to fame through the years has been caring for trauma patients," says the 53-year-old, award-winning administrator, who also happens to be the first African-American female in Detroit history to rise from the rank of Registered Nurse to hospital president.

"At the same time, we're determined to continue building our record for excellence in several other areas of research and treatment, such as hypertension, diabetes and gerontology."

Dragged from a Blazing Tanker Truck

Driver survived
horrendous burn injury

When they brought the injured truck driver into the Burn Center at Detroit Receiving Hospital, he was at the point of death. At least half his body had been severely burned by gasoline flames after the chemical-laden truck he'd been driving crashed head-on into a bridge abutment. Even worse, the unfortunate driver had breathed in some of the red-hot gases released by the roaring inferno created by the explosion.

Dr. Michael T. White, director of Detroit Receiving Hospital's Burn Center, remembers that autumn afternoon in 2004.

"At first glance, things looked pretty grim," recalls the 40-year-old general surgeon, who specializes in treating burn injuries with "Hyperbaric Oxygen Therapy" in which damaged tissues are flooded with pure oxygen in a specially designed, high-pressure chamber. "Unfortunately, the driver of the chemical truck had been burned over more than 50 percent of his body.

"He was also suffering from a horrendous inhalation injury. His lungs were very bad, and we put him on a ventilator immediately. This patient went on to spend more than two months in critical condition, and things didn't seem promising for a very long time.

"The patient was unresponsive for weeks. After months of therapy, including dozens of sessions in our hyperbaric chamber, the driver went home and rejoined his family," recalls White. "These days, he's back at work and continuing his therapy as an outpatient."

Describing the goals of the highly specialized unit, which cares for about

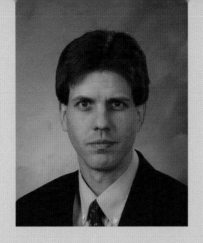

"When I look back on cases like that one, I really feel encouraged about our ability to provide the very best burn-injury treatment available in the U.S."

- Michael T. White, M.D.

350 burn victims from across the Midwest, Dr. White points out that saving the truck driver required "a great deal of determination and endurance" on the part of the custom-tailored medical team that looked after the patient. "That case speaks volumes about the outstanding care provided by our treatment teams," he says proudly. "That patient presented all of us with a real endurance test, and it was quite thrilling to eventually send him home after such a brutal and disabling injury."

Hyperbaric Therapy: A Detroit Receiving Hospital First

A general surgeon who earned his M.D. at the Wayne State University School of Medicine (1990), Mike White says he relishes the challenge involved in caring for burn patients, who often require months of arduous medical treatment and rehabilitation therapy before they can resume their shattered lives.

"I probably spend about 60 percent of my time as a surgeon working with burn patients," says the Kalamazoo native and widely published medical researcher.

"The critical care aspects of treating burn patients are extremely interesting because you usually have to sit down and map out a very complex plan of surgeries and other therapies in order to arrive at your final goal of the best possible outcome for the patient."

One of the most helpful weapons against burn-injury in the DMC's arsenal is Hyperbaric Oxygen Therapy, or HBOT. "For many patients, HBOT can be a hugely important step on the road to recovery," says the DMC specialist. Detroit Receiving Hospital's Burn Center was the first facility in the U.S. to employ

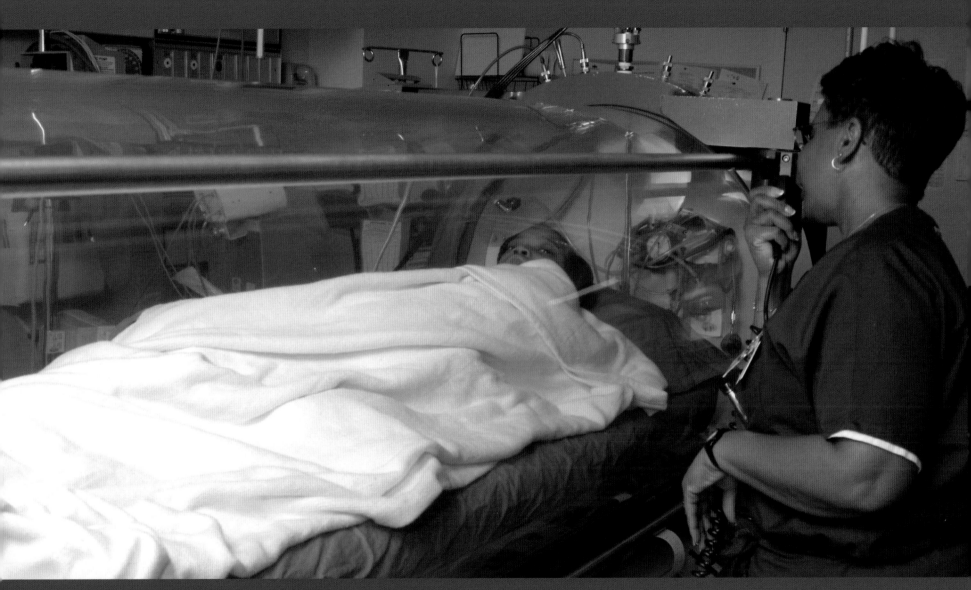

Hyperbaric Oxygen Therapy is a non-invasive, painless procedure that lasts about 90 minutes.

this exciting new technology as a treatment for burns, smoke inhalation and other medical conditions.

HBOT is the way to put pure oxygen at the site of a burn or wound. Because oxygen is under pressure two or three times greater than normal atmospheric pressure, the healing gas is forced deep into affected tissues.

The therapy enhances the bacteria-killing power of the body's white blood cells.

"HBOT also stimulates the growth of new blood cells," Dr. White explains, "which helps to boost the human body's own natural system for healing exposed wounds and burns."

Patients who undergo the treatment are usually pleased to learn that it causes little or no discomfort, and that they can move around comfortably inside the spacious chamber. Fewer than five percent will experience minor side effects, which can include the kind of irritating but harmless ear and sinus discomfort often experienced during airplane travel.

"HBOT has been recognized as a successful 'adjunctive' treatment for burns and other medical conditions," says Dr. White, "and the therapy has been endorsed by such authoritative organizations as the American Medical Association and Medicare in addition to many commercial health insurers."

Dr. White concludes, "As a pioneer in the use of this powerful new healing tool, we're standing at the forefront of an effort to provide burn patients with the latest and best technologies available in the world."

"As a pioneer in the use of this powerful new healing tool, we're standing at the forefront of an effort to provide burn patients with the latest and best technologies available in the world."

— Michael T. White, M.D.

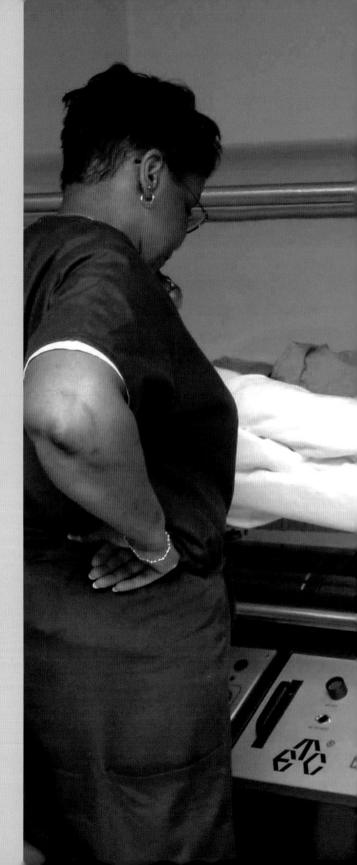

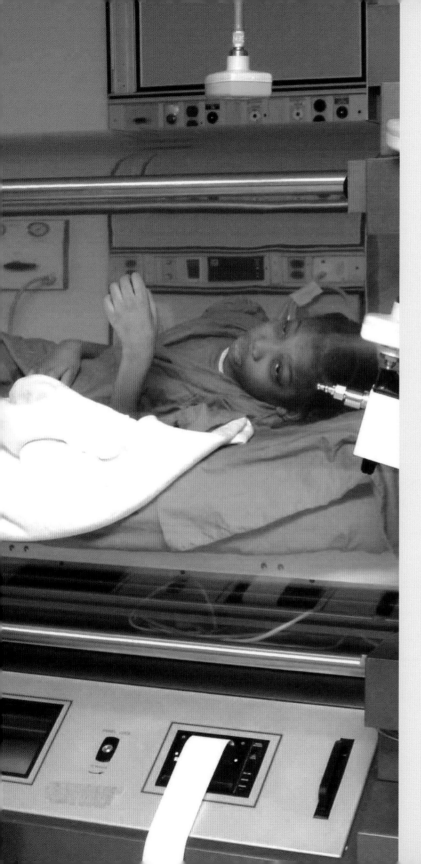

Establishing a world-class trauma center

Question: Ever wondered how many medical patients visit the DMC's Emergency Department at Receiving Hospital each year?

Answer: More than 80,000.

Question: How about the adjoining University Health Center (UHC) where Wayne State University-based health care professionals operate more than two dozen clinics for outpatients from all across southeast Michigan?

Answer: The Center treats more than 250,000 Michiganders yearly.

So what's it like to run these two huge urban medical complexes on a daily basis?

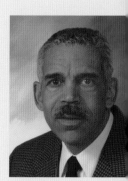

Leslie C. Bowman

"Challenging!" says Leslie C. Bowman, the former President of the DMC's Receiving Hospital and UHC, who retired in 2004 after more than 23 years as a high-level administrator at Michigan's largest and busiest medical center.

"I started working at Receiving back in 1978 when it was still known as the old 'Detroit General,'" explains the 66-year-old Bowman, who put in nearly two decades as Receiving's Chief Operating Officer before taking the helm as President there in the late 1990s. "For those of us who were running the hospital, that period was extremely challenging and difficult because we were right in the middle of moving the entire complex from downtown to its present location on the DMC campus at midtown.

"Was it a tough assignment? You bet. But I was thrilled to be part of it because, from the very beginning, I really loved the mission of Receiving Hospital, which was to provide the very best trauma and emergency medicine in Michigan."

For Bowman, an easygoing and congenial administrator with a knack for recruiting talented managers, one of the "biggest breakthroughs" in trauma care at Receiving took place in 1987 when the American College of Surgeons (ACS) awarded "Verified" status to the facility's trauma-care program. That early designation marked Receiving as only the second hospital in the United States to receive such a trauma-program verification by the ACS.

"For most of us at Receiving that was a thrilling moment," says Bowman today. "It took years of continuing effort to build the training program up to that level of performance. We were proud of meeting the challenge."

"New frontier" in skull-replacement surgery

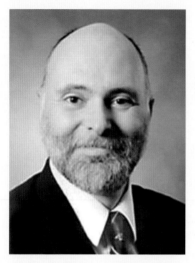

Daniel B. Michael, M.D., Ph.D.

He was the first neurosurgeon in the world to repair a human skull with a recently invented substance known as "bionic bone."

It happened back in the spring of 2000 during a widely reported neurosurgery operation at Detroit Receiving Hospital.

Ask 50-year-old Daniel B. Michael, M.D., to remember the moment when he and a team of DMC surgeons made medical history, and this highly regarded surgeon won't mince his words. "I do think we crossed an important frontier that day," says the high-voltage Dr. Michael, an extraordinarily creative physician who plays the bass in a Motown rock band when he isn't performing brain surgery or teaching at the Wayne State University School of Medicine.

"Our skull-repair procedure was the first one in which surgeons used a substance that allows new bone to grow into it rather than employing the traditional steel or titanium plate, which can never be 'fitted' exactly to the patient's own unique skull structure.

"For those of us who worked on the project at Detroit Receiving, that first step toward a 'bionic skull implant' was quite thrilling. But it was only the beginning, really. I expect that five or 10 years down the road, we're going to be seeing some amazing things in the area of bio-materials for skull and neurological surgery alike."

A tall, powerfully built figure who sports a rakish goatee, Dr. Michael has earned a growing reputation in recent years as a brain surgeon who loves to "push the envelope" by designing new materials and inventing sophisticated new brain-injury computer models aimed at radically improving the art of neurosurgery.

Known as "bone source cranioplasty," Dr. Michael's unique approach to "filling in" missing segments of the injured skull is technically complex but easy to explain as a medical concept.

In most cases, he says, the procedure takes place after the surgeon prepares a flexible, putty-like substance, "hydroxyapaptite," and then applies it to traumatized areas of the skull where bone loss has occurred.

Using highly accurate 3-D computer tomography (CT) technology, the gifted neurosurgeon then shapes an exact "mold" that duplicates the missing bone segment. After application, the special putty congeals to form a rock-like substance that then allows human bone to grow deeply into it. Eventually, the patient's new skull bone merges with the putty to completely restore the missing skull segment.

As several U.S. medical journals have noted in recent years, the process offers two huge advantages to most skull-trauma patients.

First, the "bionic bone implant" eliminates the need for "harvesting" new skull bone from the patient's hip, thus eliminating the hazards and discomforts that would be involved in a second surgery.

Second, Dr. Michael's approach to cranioplasty greatly reduces the chances of infection in the affected areas of the skull since the bionic bone is microscopically sterile from the beginning.

The enormous promise contained in this new, state-of-the-art technology became evident back in 2000 when Dr. Michael and his Detroit Receiving colleagues first used it on a 41-year-old Detroit mom who'd lost part of the frontal and temporal areas of her skull to a bone infection after undergoing brain surgery to repair an aneuryism.

Reported by CNN, the Associated Press and several major newspapers, the successful, first-of-its-kind operation completely eliminated the "caved-in" appearance of the patient's damaged skull within less than a year. After being forced to wear an injury-hiding scarf for several years, the grateful patient was able to dispense with the camouflage and forget about her former disfigurement entirely. Since that initial operation, Dr. Michael's new technique has been adopted by dozens of brain surgeons all across the country.

How important is Dr. Michael's surgical breakthrough for brain-injury patients in the United States today?

"If you look at the current data, you'll find that more than 50,000 Americans die each year because of trauma or disease that destroys a portion of the skull," says the widely published Wayne State University Medical School graduate, who grew up in the Detroit area as the science-loving son of a General Motors chemical engineer. "At the same time, another two million brain-injury patients will lose some degree of vital functioning because of skull-related trauma and disease.

"As a brain surgeon, I consider those numbers to be a national tragedy," says the Detroit Receiving Chief of Neurosurgery and Wayne State medical professor, who also owns a Ph.D. in anatomy and cell biology. "That's why we're working night and day to make this new cranioplasty procedure available to every brain-surgery unit in the country.

"When you think about how these new kinds of surgical techniques are going to benefit patients all around the globe, you can't wait to get into the hospital each morning."

"When you think about how these new kinds of surgical techniques are going to benefit patients all around the globe, you can't wait to get into the hospital each morning."

- Daniel B. Michael, M.D., Ph.D.

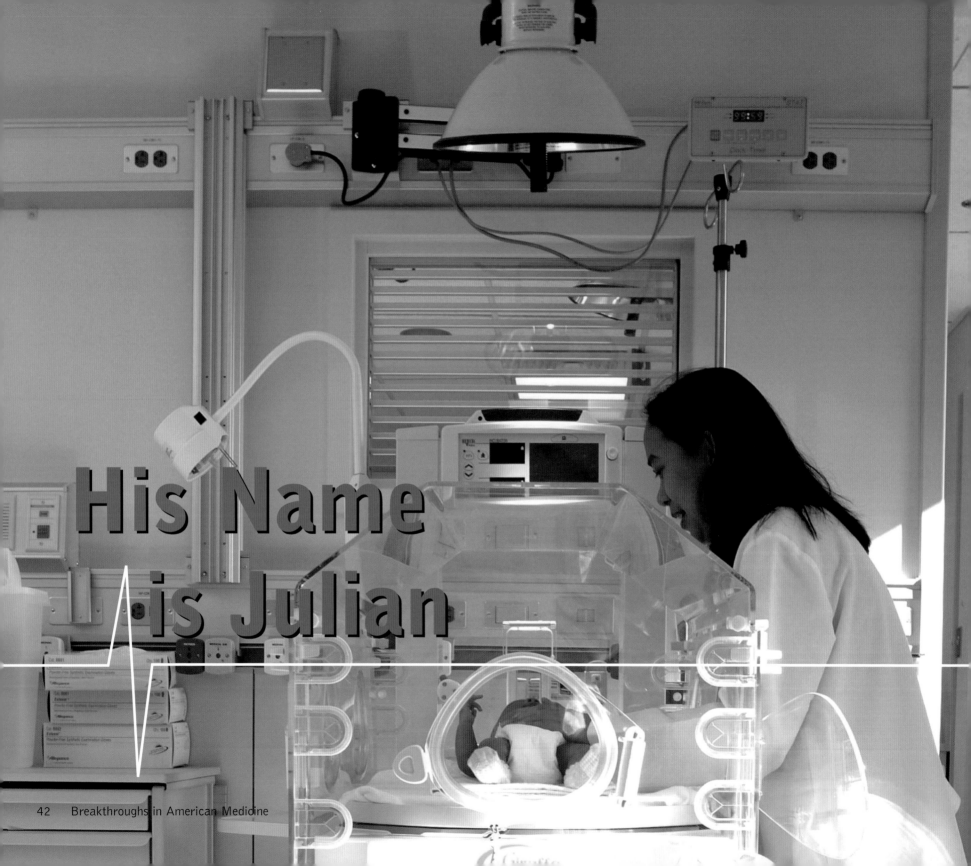

His Name
is Julian

High-tech neonatal intensive-care unit battles to save one-pound baby's life

His name is Julian Gabriel Moulton English, and he came into the world on a bitterly cold day in January 2004. On the day he was born at Detroit's Hutzel Women's Hospital, Julian weighed slightly more than one pound.

Like 400,000 other U.S. newborns each year, he was premature — a potentially life-threatening condition in which birth occurs before the 37th week of gestation.

The number of such premature births has been growing rapidly in America during the past two decades, to the point that one childbirth in 10 now takes place earlier than it should. (The national price tag for this spiraling epidemic is $5 billion per year.)

Because Julian had arrived more than 14 weeks early, the chances for his survival seemed slim.

The battle that lay ahead — literally a battle for Julian's life — would be long and exhausting, and it would require thousands of hours of dedicated work by the doctors, nurse practitioners and staff nurses, discharge coordinators, respiratory therapists, pharmacists, radiologists and chaplains who are part of the Hutzel Neonatal Intensive Care Unit (NICU) team.

As the long days unfolded and Julian's life hung in the balance, the NICU team worked diligently to save him. One key member of that team is nurse manager Rosalyn Hall. Armed with three different nursing degrees and 36 years of nursing experience, the 55-year-old Hall is officially described as the "Director of Patient Care Services" at the Hutzel NICU and Special Care Nursery. A veteran professional, the soft-spoken and cheerful Hall supervises more than 100 nurses and support staff who typically care for 18-20 premature babies each day. Using state-of-the-art technology — including the world's only nursery-based "Micro-Positron Emission Tomography (PET) Scanner" — Hall's NICU has established a long track record as one of the most effective neonatal treatment centers in the world.

Make no mistake: In the struggle to keep little Julian alive, the NICU would be fully tested.

Located on the third floor of the sprawling Hutzel Women's

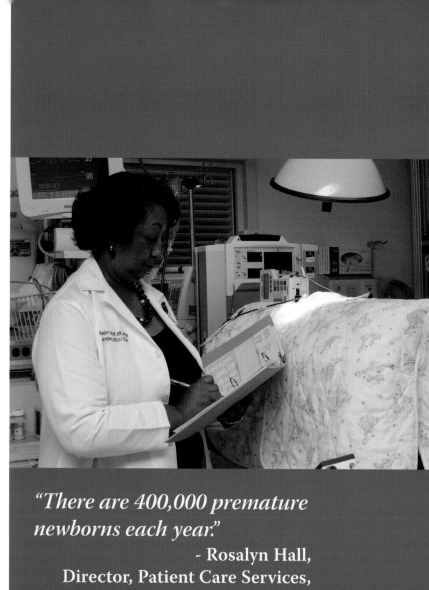

"There are 400,000 premature newborns each year."

**- Rosalyn Hall,
Director, Patient Care Services,
Hutzel Women's Hospital**

Hospital in midtown Detroit, the NICU is a vast, swarming facility with 36 neonatal intensive-care beds and a mind-bending array of high-tech equipment designed to keep struggling infants alive and breathing.

That last word — "breathing" — is the key to everything that goes on in the NICU, according to Hall.

"The most important thing to understand about premature babies is that their little lungs aren't fully developed," she said one day recently while describing the long campaign to save Julian's life. "When an infant is born more than 14 weeks early, and weighs little more than a pound, you're going to have multiple health problems, including respiratory issues, infections and nutritional and developmental problems."

After Julian was stabilized, the NICU team placed him on a ventilator. But immaturity of the lungs was only one of the dangers he faced now. Because his skin was also immature and undeveloped, he would also be vulnerable to a wide array of pathogens — life-threatening bacterial and viral microorganisms that cause multiple infections, placing his life in jeopardy.

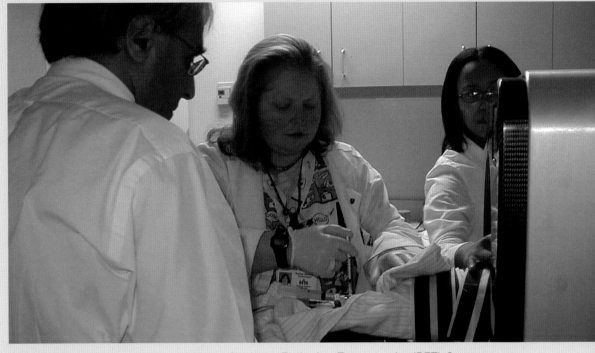

The world's only nursery-based Micro-Positron Emission Tomography (PET) Scanner.

To combat infections, the NICU team would pump a steady supply of antibiotics into Julian's bloodstream — powerful allies, fed into his system by an intravenous ("IV") catheter, that would boost his ability to fend off the growing ranks of microscopic attackers.

So far, so good. But what about nutrition? Because of his immature digestive system, the NICU team was challenged to feed Julian nutrients that would help

him to grow and develop. To accomplish that, they would have to employ a special feeding tube.

Problems, problems. "Another key issue for premature babies is blood pressure," says Roz Hall, who's been running the Hutzel NICU for the past 15 years. "A premature baby's blood pressure tends to fluctuate, and one of our strategies for coping with that is dopamine, a medication designed to steady and strengthen the heartbeat. Julian received a dopamine drip to help maintain his blood pressure."

Once the NICU team succeeded in stabilizing Julian, they settled in for the long haul. During the next 10 weeks or so, they would participate in a grueling endurance race — an hour-by-hour marathon that required endless, careful vigilance and instant reaction at the first sign of a health complication linked to the child's compromised metabolic and circulatory systems.

"As always, the NICU team did a terrific job of monitoring the baby and responding with timely interventions when required," says Hall. "These are some wonderful people! They hang in there night and day, doing everything they can to support the infants and families in our care.

"They will give you 100 percent, every single time. I've seen them work 16 hours at a stretch without complaint in order to make sure that every baby we have receives the very best care. They give their best — even on the days when things aren't going so well, the days when you have a baby turn toward the worst, or the days when you're losing a baby and it's the seventh time the mother has tried and failed to have a child, and once again,

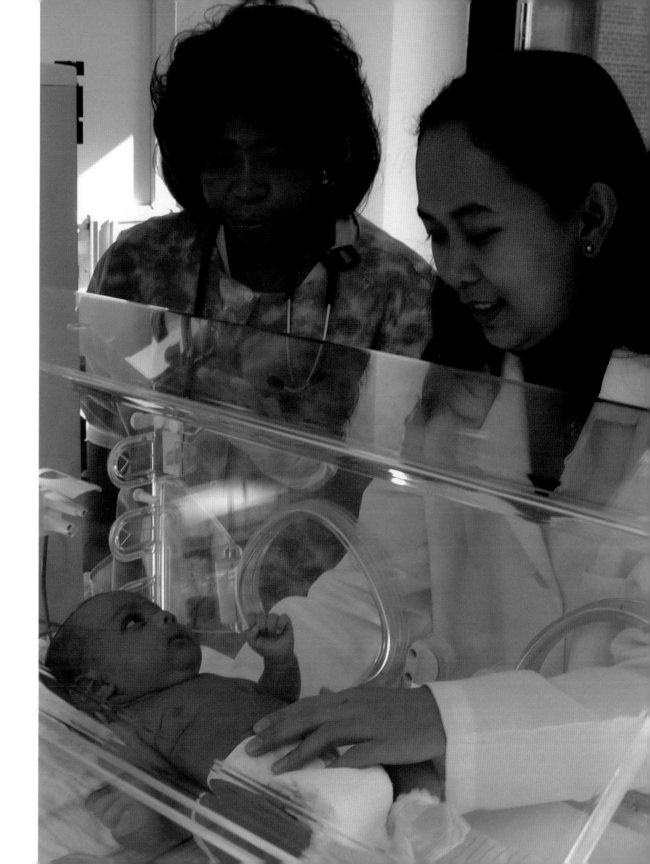

you're going to have to give her the bad news.

"It's tough. But these are the most dedicated people I've ever met. I've got nurses on this unit who've worked here 25 and 30 years. I've even got one who's been here 35 years! You talk about dedication and commitment? I truly mean it when I say: I could not work with a better group of people."

As the weeks passed and Baby Julian slowly grew stronger, the NICU team was also able to take advantage of an innovation unique to the DMC. Originally invented in order to study the internal organs of tiny laboratory animals, the "Micro-PET Scanner" has, for several years, been employed by DMC Children's Hospital physician Harry Chugani, M.D., as an invaluable tool that allows specialists to check premature infants for neurological abnormalities caused by their early births.

Armed with state-of-the-art monitoring devices, the NICU staffers were able to keep a watchful eye over every aspect of Baby Julian's growth. As the weeks passed and the tiny infant continued to gain weight, the members of the team felt increasingly hopeful about the eventual outcome.

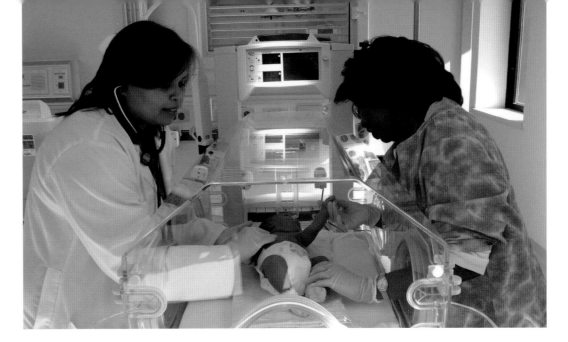

"75 percent of the morbidity and mortality of babies is related to spontaneous pre-term delivery; 50 percent of infant mortality is related to premature delivery."

- Yoram Sorokin, M.D.

"After a few weeks, we were really starting to feel good about Julian's chances," says Hall today. "But we never take anything for granted in the NICU, because things can change very quickly, kind of like a roller coaster. There are days on which it seems like every baby in Detroit is delivering at Hutzel and every baby is premature!"

A devout Baptist who often works with church-linked ministries that supply her NICU with hundreds of donated bonnets, booties, gowns and other baby items each year, Roz Hall says she also relies on the "spiritual comfort" she obtains from a special prayer she long ago attached to her office door. Among other things, that eloquent prayer asks for help in coping with the "terrific stress" that often accompanies work on a neonatal ICU.

O Lord, even in this day's most stressful hour, may I rest in the peace and perfection of Your healing Presence. . .

After more than 15 weeks of diligent, around-the-clock medical care, little Julian departed the NICU with his beaming mother late in the summer of 2004. The hard-working NICU team took a well-deserved deep breath before turning back to the other infants in their care.

One year later, on a bright summer morning in the Motor City, Julian returned with his mother for a brief visit to the unit where his life had begun.

"As I looked at him, I felt pretty good," says Rosalyn Hall. "As a matter of fact, I felt very good. That really lifts your spirits when they come back to the NICU for a 'thank-you visit' and you see the happy parents playing with their precious child.

"I wouldn't work at any other place!"

Added the happy mom, Natasha Moulton-Levy, a professional health care consultant who now lives in Maryland: "Julian is walking very well. He has also started saying words now that he has hearing aids to overcome the hearing loss he suffered from his prematurity. Obviously, I'm thrilled and immensely pleased by the outcome in his case, and I really mean it when I say: I love Hutzel Hospital.

"I'm very grateful to the doctors and all the nurses like Roz Hall who fought so hard to keep my son alive so that I could take him home, watch him grow and love him the way I do today!"

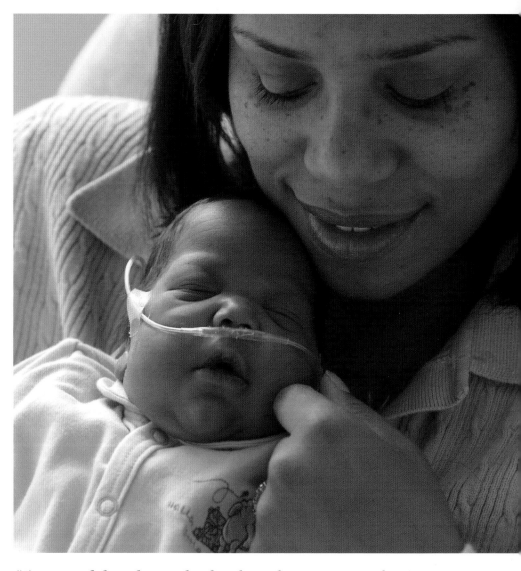

"I'm grateful to those who fought to keep my son alive."

- Natasha Moulton-Levy

The future looked childless until the high-risk pregnancy unit arrived

After struggling through six consecutive miscarriages, the young married couple from West Bloomfield had nearly despaired.

But then they got a nice surprise.

At the DMC's Hutzel Women's Hospital, a high-risk pregnancy specialist named Dr. Marjorie Treadwell answered their plaintive question — *Should we give up?* — with a single, ringing word: "No!" Instead of recommending that Chris and Maria Xiromeritis abandon their decade-long quest for a baby, the Director of Obstetric Ultrasound suggested a series of state-of-the-art blood tests.

And that's when the grieving couple finally got a break.

It happened when Dr. Treadwell's tests disclosed that a genetic mutation had triggered abnormal functioning in a key protein linked to fetal development during all six of Maria's miscarriages.

Known medically as a "MTHFR mutation," the disorder can cause stillbirth, miscarriage or even birth defects. But Dr. Treadwell also noted that this condition can often be treated successfully with folic acid to boost protein for healthy fetal growth.

After a detailed medical evaluation by Dr. Treadwell, Maria began taking the substance. With their hopes revived, the couple decided on yet another attempt at having a child.

What followed was a tense journey through a difficult pregnancy. Uneasy and alarmed much of the time, the gutsy couple hung on day by day while drawing "enormous strength" and lots of helpful advice from the supportive physician.

"Dr. Treadwell was terrific," Maria recalls today. "She did ultrasounds on me weekly, and she had a knack for pinpointing issues related to my pregnancy. Her expert use of the ultrasound was especially helpful in meeting all of the developing baby's needs."

After months of suspense, an ecstatic Maria Xiromeritis gave birth to a premature, but healthy daughter, Ava, in the spring of 2004.

Says Dr. Treadwell, while describing that happy event: "When you wind up with an outcome like that one, there's obviously a feeling of great satisfaction on the part of everyone involved. I really do believe we have one of the best ultrasound units at work in this country today."

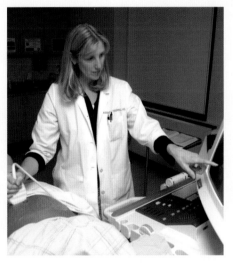

Marjorie Treadwell, M.D.

But the story of Chris and Maria and Ava doesn't end there.

Shortly before this book went to press, a delighted Maria Xiromeritis announced that she was once again expecting — and that she was already 30 weeks into her *next* healthy pregnancy.

"We're expecting our second daughter, Zoe, to join us within a few months, and so far, everything has been going very well," said the joyful mother-to-be.

"We think Dr. Treadwell is awesome — and we're 'DMC all the way!'"

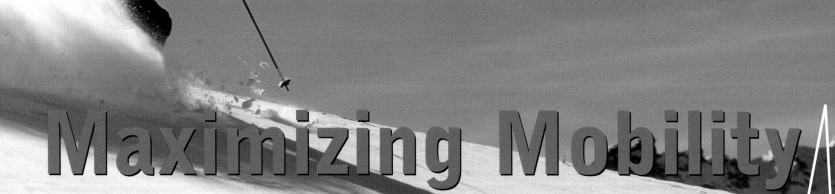

Maximizing Mobility

Who says you can't ''hit the slopes''after getting knee-replacement surgery?

Before his recent knee-replacement surgery, 77-year-old Conrad Mallett Sr., loved to zoom down challenging ski slopes from New England to Colorado.

Whether he was soaring over a three-foot high mogul or kicking up a blizzard of powdery snow as he spun through a high-powered turn, the highly athletic Mr. Mallett — the father of former Michigan Supreme Court Justice Conrad Mallett Jr. — continued to enjoy his favorite sport, long after retirement.

But during the summer of 2004, advancing age finally began to catch up with this high-flying septuagenarian after painful arthritis in both knees left him increasingly unable to don his skis and attack the slopes.

Was Mallett's career as a downhill blade-runner finished?

Amazingly enough, the answer turned out to be *no*. Determined to hang onto his skiing ability, Mallett opted for "artificial knees" — completely new joints that were recently installed during state-of-the-art, "minimally invasive" surgery at the DMC's Sinai-Grace Hospital.

After undergoing the two knee-replacement procedures in 2004, the feisty Mallett soon began to recover his athletic skills. He immediately started planning brand-new skiing expeditions to the Berkshire Mountains of New England and the Rocky Mountains of the west.

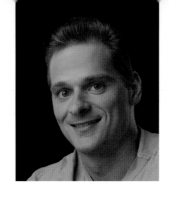

"We can greatly reduce the amount of discomfort the patient experiences and also dramatically reduce recovery time."

- Robert Ference, M.D.

"I won't be skiing any 'expert' slopes at my age," he says with a chuckle, "but it's good to know that I *will* be able to remain active on the slopes, thanks to the innovative knee-replacement surgery I received at Sinai-Grace!"

The new Sinai-Grace procedure allows more than 96 percent of the patients who receive Dr. Ference's procedure to resume their normal activities in between two and six weeks compared to the three-to-six-months of recovery time required for the traditional knee replacement surgery.

Currently, Sinai-Grace is the only hospital offering Dr. Ference's modified, even less invasive version of the "minimally invasive knee-replacement surgery."

The highly regarded orthopaedic surgeon Robert Ference, M.D. has already conducted nearly 900 of his modified minimally invasive surgeries. His reaction? "Although I've done hundreds of these knee-replacements, I'm still astonished when I see the results," Dr. Ference says today. "By making tiny incisions and avoiding trauma to the muscles that surround the knee such as the quadriceps or thigh muscles, we can greatly reduce the amount of discomfort the patient experiences and also dramatically reduce recovery time."

According to Dr. Ference, his version of this minimally invasive procedure requires far less recovery time and far less pain than traditional knee-replacement surgery for three key reasons:

• the surgeon makes a knee incision of only three or four inches, compared to the 12-inch incision that often occurs in traditional knee-replacement surgery.

• the surgeon doesn't cut into the all-important quadriceps muscle, which was an essential step in the traditional method as well as in the traditional minimally invasive technique. Great effort also is taken to be as gentle to the surrounding muscles and tissues of the knee.

• the doctor only lifts the kneecap slightly from the underlying bone structure without flipping it over as required with the older method.

Dr. Ference is also quick to point out his knee replacement team always takes "extraordinary measures" to prevent infection from taking place during or after a surgical procedure. Those precautions include the preparation of special "antibiotic cement" that is used to hold the implants and that provides structural support for artificial knees. Dr. Ference and his colleagues wear "bubble suits" with space-age-looking helmets and special surgical gowns during all surgical procedures involving knee replacement. These precautions help him maintain an infection rate of 0.02% — which is astonishing.

"This new knee replacement method is one of the most exciting things I've seen in my orthopeadic practice," says the upbeat Dr. Ference, who has brought national attention to Sinai-Grace —

along with hundreds of patients from all across the country and internationally — because of his pioneering work in outfitting patients with brand new knees. "I can assure you it's very rewarding and very gratifying to have patients tell you they 'can't believe' how quickly they recovered from their total knee-replacement surgery.

"We've had people come to the DMC from California to Connecticut and from Texas to Canada. And now, even Poland. I think this kind of track record shows people really understand the desirability of a 'minimally invasive' approach to surgery."

Because the new procedure uses much smaller instruments and affects far less tissue than past procedures, "Just about anybody who needs a knee replacement or revision is a good candidate," says the veteran DMC orthopeadist. "In addition, today's knee replacements are expected to last from 20 to 30 years — which makes them quite

suitable for a wide range of age groups.

"Here at Sinai-Grace, we've done knee replacements for patients from age 24 to age 94, and for patients who weighed from 150 pounds to 415 pounds. And we can help patients who are struggling with conditions that range from arthritis to severe deformities."

Recently, Dr. Ference has added computer navigation to his technique. Patients, who once were not candidates for minimally invasive surgery because of previous hardware in bones around the knee or severe deformity of the leg bones, are now able to benefit from his innovative approach. Computer navigation further aids in measuring to assure every step of the surgery is perfect.

"If chronic knee pain is affecting your life and limiting your ability to do the things you enjoy, you may very well be a candidate for our rapidly expanding program at the DMC," exclaims Dr. Ference.

"If chronic knee pain is affecting your life and limiting your ability to do the things you enjoy, you may very well be a candidate for our rapidly expanding program at the DMC."

- Robert Ference, M.D.

Innovative new "reverse shoulder" technique saves arthritis patients from "a life of pain"

When the 83-year-old arthritis victim finally called out for help, she was in so much pain that she couldn't raise her right arm — not even to lift a fork at the dinner table.

Like tens of thousands of other senior citizens on any given day in America, this troubled senior citizen was struggling with a disabling condition in which severe shoulder arthritis — combined with a torn "rotator cuff" joint — caused her agonizing pain, even as it severely restricted her arm movement.

Until quite recently, patients like this one were usually told that surgery could not improve their condition — with little promising relief of their pain and no improvement in their ability to use their arm.

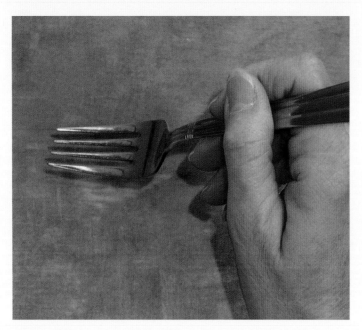

But that's not what happened to the independent-minded senior citizen from the Detroit suburb of Roseville, in the spring of 2005. Instead of resigning herself to a life of limited mobility and increasing discomfort, this feisty senior decided to educate herself about the latest, state-of-the-art medical procedure aimed at replacing defective shoulder joints like hers.

After several weeks of diligent research, she wound up paying a visit to one of the nation's most experienced and innovative arthritis specialists — Dr. Steve Petersen, an award-winning surgeon at the Detroit Medical Center's Michigan Orthopaedic Specialty Hospital (MIOSH), Associate Professor and Acting Chairman of Wayne State University School of Medicine, Department of Orthopaedic Surgery.

Fortunately for the Roseville resident, Dr. Petersen is one of the country's founding practitioners of a remarkable new medical procedure known as "reverse shoulder surgery," in which the surgeon repairs the damaged shoulder by inserting a new "ball-and-socket" mechanism that reverses the natural position of both, and then mechanically improves the ability to move his/her arm painlessly.

After assembling a detailed patient history and conducting a thorough physical exam, the DMC specialist concluded that his new patient was an appropriate candidate for the promising, high-tech procedure.

And the outcome? "For this patient, the results were very positive and life-changing," says Dr. Petersen, who has performed the operation more than 20 times during the past few years. "Within a few weeks, this delighted senior was able to lift her arm to eye level and then fully extend it, without any discernible pain at all. As you might imagine, this improvement in range of motion gave her a huge boost.

"For elderly arthritis-sufferers like this one, being able to feed yourself and attend to other essential tasks of daily life provides a great deal of independence and flexibility. These days, she's free to live an active, vigorous life entirely on her own.

"As a physician and an orthopaedic surgeon, I take a great deal of satisfaction from outcomes like this one because they can be so hugely important when it comes to improving the quality of life and mobility of patients."

Designed specifically for patients who struggle with shoulder arthritis and a torn rotator cuff, the innovative new procedure is unique in the way that it "reverses" the position of the ball and the socket in shoulder anatomy. Recently approved by the FDA, for the very specific indication of rotator cuff arthropathy,

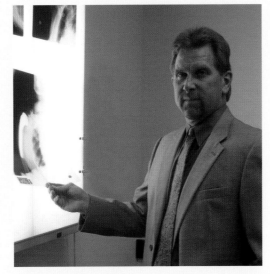

Steve Petersen, M.D.

the procedure has been drawing rave reviews around the country from patients who say that it eliminates most of the severe pain that occurs in cases where "bone rubs against bone" after structural damage caused by severe arthritis with associated irreparable rotator cuff tearing.

"After helping so many patients with the new procedure, I'm convinced that it's going to become an important new surgical option in the years immediately up ahead," says Dr.

Petersen, a veteran orthopaedic surgeon who, as the Chief of Orthopaedic Surgery at MIOSH, is a nationally recognized shoulder specialist. "There's no doubt that reverse shoulder surgery is here to stay, or that it's going to make a major difference in the lives of many seniors.

"I also believe that this exciting new surgery is a perfect example of the kind of innovative clinical care that has made the Michigan Orthopaedic Hospital a national leader in arthritis care during recent years."

Adds the highly regarded DMC clinician and health researcher: "Although a lot of people don't realize it, arthritis patients live with an enormous burden of pain and discomfort, day in and day out. All too often, that discomfort leads to immobility and then a withdrawal from the normal activities of life. This can be followed by depression and frequently a decline in quality of life.

"For a physician, helping to alter that scenario by performing this kind of innovative surgery is an exciting opportunity to serve patients well. It's also a big part of the reason why I can't wait to get into work each day!"

The First Steps, Again

Unique program stresses
spinal cord recovery

Cortney Hoffman doesn't remember what happened during the auto accident or during the terrible hours that immediately followed it.

For Cortney — an attractive, 19-year-old resident of small-town Temperance, Michigan — the memory of her 2002 car crash ends with the sounds of screaming tires and shattering glass. But she says she will never forget the days that followed the disaster, agonizing days in which she lived with the despair of being told that her spinal cord had been crushed and that she would probably never walk again.

"When the doctors explained what had happened to me, I was absolutely devastated," says Cortney today. "As a kid, I'd loved playing all kinds of different sports, and I'd always been very active. And now, I was suddenly looking at a future in which I wouldn't even be able to walk to the grocery store.

"At first, I got really down. I nearly gave up. I felt totally depressed, and I didn't know if I'd have the strength to endure life in a wheelchair."

Although she'd been unlucky behind the wheel — to say the least — Cortney's future began to look much brighter after she learned from the news media about a uniquely innovative program at the DMC's Rehabilitation Institute of Michigan (RIM). That RIM program, directed by a nationally renowned expert on spinal cord injury Dr. Steven Hinderer,

Detroit Free Press

METRO FINAL
50 cents

www.freep.com

STEM CELL MEDICINE | HELP FOR PARALYSIS

Cortney's wish is to walk again

Teen to undergo innovative surgery

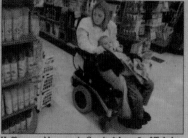

Hoffman and her cousin Cassie Adney, 5, of Toledo shop last week at a dollar store.

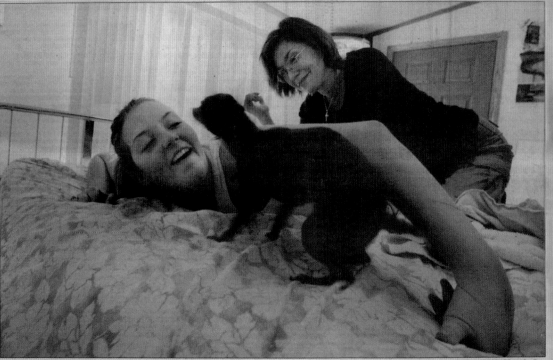

Photos by ERIC SEALS/Detroit Free Press

Tika, a 3-year-old Chihuahua, visits as Cortney Hoffman, 18, of Temperance gets a massage last week from her therapist Kristie Tellier, 46, of Hillsdale. Hoffman was paralyzed from the chest down after a car accident in July 2002. On Saturday, she'll undergo stem-cell surgery that she hopes will help her walk.

By PATRICIA ANSTETT
FREE PRESS MEDICAL WRITER

Cortney Hoffman admits the painful truth. She wasn't wearing a seat belt the day her car flew off the road less than a month after she received her driver's license on her 16th birthday.

She was just going a few miles to her cousin's house. She insists she wasn't speeding, sleepy, drunk or stoned, but she has no idea how her 1996 Cutlass Supreme landed in a ditch on July 30, 2002.

She recalls calling for help from the ditch after being thrown from her car on a freshly resurfaced gravel road.

About 10 minutes later, a man driving by heard her muffled plea, followed her voice, found her and called for help.

Hoffman awoke in a Toledo hospital, paralyzed from her shoulders down.

Six days later, she was told she'd never walk again.

Today, she departs on a plane to Lisbon, Portugal, for experimental stem-cell surgery Saturday.

Her goal is to walk at her own wedding some day. "I'm not getting married until I can walk down the aisle by myself," said Hoffman, an upbeat 18-year-old from Temperance, north of Toledo,

who likes to hunt, sing and shop, particularly for jewelry. She is 5 feet, 6 inches tall with bright blue eyes and blonde hair, a 21st-Century version of the girl next door, with a big smile and ear piercings.

Her strongest attributes are an upbeat personality and persistence, said her mother, Tammi Roe, a divorcee who lives with her daughter. She quit her job as a furniture maker to take care of Cortney after the accident.

"She always has a smile on her face every day," Roe said. "She has just

Please see STEM CELLS, Page 8A

MORE IN BODY & MIND

Meet Erica Nader of Farmington Hills, the first American to undergo the Portuguese stem-cell procedure. She's making progress. **6H**

AND COMING FRIDAY: Cortney Hoffman travels to Portugal to prepare for her stem-cell surgery.

MONDAY: Cortney undergoes the 5-hour experimental surgery.

TUESDAY: Will the procedure work? If it does, her paralyzed limbs should feel warm and tingly within 24 hours.

is the first hospital-based program in the nation to focus on "recovery," rather than mere "therapeutic rehabilitation," from severe spinal cord injury.

"What's really unique about our program is that word recovery," says the widely published specialist at RIM. "In most spinal cord injury programs around the country, the emphasis is on teaching patients how to 'adjust' to the kinds of injuries that leave them wheelchair bound.

"But our philosophy at RIM is completely different, and our entire approach is based on recovering from injuries, not merely learning how to live with them.

"At RIM, we take a uniquely 'aggressive' approach to therapy. Our workout sessions last longer, for example, and they usually demand as much as possible from patients. Our treatment model is based on athletic-training procedures that emphasize friendly competition and self-motivation.

"I think the good news for spinal cord patients everywhere is that we're already seeing very positive results with this 'recovery approach.' Our patients tend to regain more of their mobility and greater use of affected limbs than patients in more traditional programs that focus on merely adjusting to injuries."

For Cortney Hoffman, the outcome so far has been nothing less than spectacular.

After joining Dr. Hinderer's program in September of 2004, she decided to participate in an experimental "stem-cell surgery" that was recently launched by Portugal's famed Dr. Carlos Lima at Hospital de Egas Moniz.

Under Dr. Hinderer's direction, Cortney traveled to Lisbon, Portugal, and became only the 37th person in the world to undergo the innovative surgery, in which specially cultured stem cells are

Independent mind dealing with injuries

Rehabilitation Institute of Michigan's nationally renowned Center for Spinal Cord Injury Recovery (CSCIR) is unique in the world for its emphasis on helping patients to begin recovering from spinal cord trauma rather than merely "adjusting" to paralyzing injuries. Says CSCIR Director Dr. Steven Hinderer: "What's different about our approach is that we don't focus exclusively on traditional rehabilitation goals; we don't restrict ourselves to merely teaching patients to compensate for lost function by using whatever physical capabilities remain with them.

"Instead, we work with the patient toward goals in recovery, using both physical rehab techniques and the latest cellular implant and injection methods, such as the newly established olfactory ensheathing glia (OEG) cell transplantation process. We're also very interested in the latest stem cell technology, and we frequently send patients around the world for treatment with these cutting-edge rehab therapies.

"Our aggressive and independent-mind approach to dealing with spinal cord injury reflects the spirit of the late [injured movie actor] Christopher Reeve, who dedicated himself to finding new methods of recovery for paralyzed patients rather than simply coaching them on how to adapt to their loss of function."

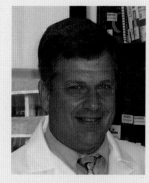

Steven Hinderer, M.D.

injected directly into the spinal cord in order to promote healing and new growth.

Along with the surgery, Cortney Hoffman began an intensive rehab program based on Dr. Hinderer's "athletic training model."

And the results? "The program demands lots of hard work," says Cortney today, "but I'm amazed at how far I've already come. Just the other day, I took my first steps in therapy — and that was a very exciting breakthrough for me! At first, a doctor told me I wouldn't ever be able to get out of bed, but now I'm up every single day, and I work out on a regular schedule.

"In addition, I'm set to enter a college degree program in speech therapy in a few months. My dream is to walk again someday. I guess I'm a lot like Christopher Reeve in that way because I know I'm not going to be content with simply 'adjusting' to my injury.

"I want to recover — and that's why I'm so glad I found a program that emphasizes recovery, here at the DMC."

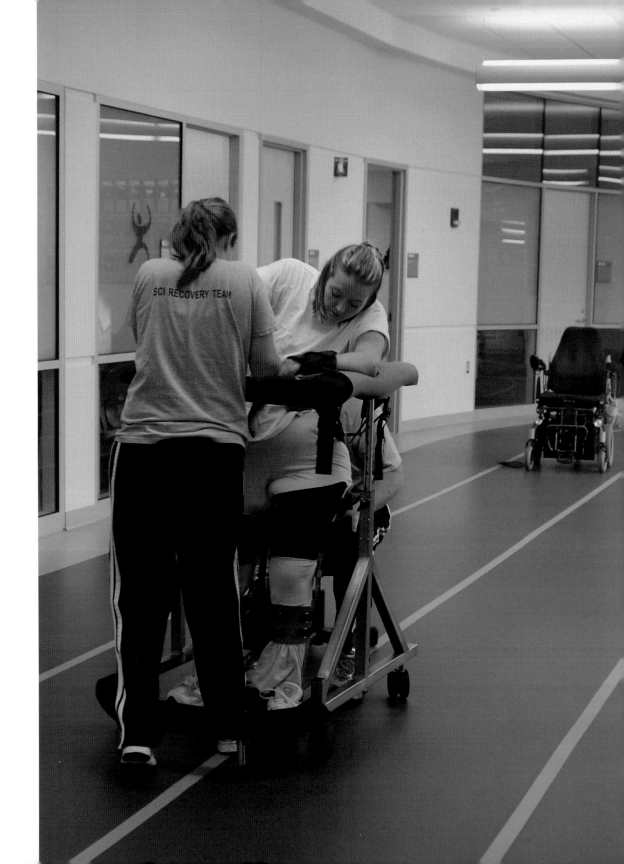

Therapist's biggest thrill, watching patients improve

He worked for 35 years as an occupational therapist at the DMC's Rehabilitation Institute of Michigan (RIM), and he says he "loved every minute of it."

Most of all, he loved it when a disabled patient under his care would learn how to function successfully again after months of grueling therapy, and then return to an active, vigorous life in his or her community.

"I spent my entire professional career as a RIM therapist," says 74-year-old Joseph Wanchik," who retired in 1993, "and during that time, I watched hundreds of patients recover from crippling injuries or illnesses and then go on to build successful lives for themselves.

"For me, there was no thrill quite like the thrill of seeing a rehab patient cope successfully with a spinal cord injury or some other disabling event. On several occasions, we had patients who improved remarkably in occupational therapy and then went on to college. One even became a successful lawyer after leaving us."

Describing one of his most exciting moments as a therapist who treated thousands

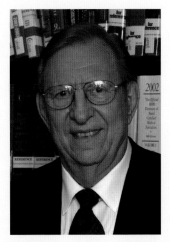

of patients through the years, the easygoing and upbeat Wanchik chuckles with nostalgia. "We created Michigan's first driver-training program for the disabled here at RIM back in the mid-1970s," he recalls, "and we built all sorts of devices to help handicapped patients turn the steering wheel or apply the brakes so they could drive an automobile safely.

"I remember one partially paralyzed patient who really struggled in order to regain the ability to drive a car. It was difficult, but he finally won the battle. And then one afternoon a few weeks later, I was driving along the Chrysler Freeway headed home from work and he passed me up!

"He zoomed right past me in his car, and it was a terrific moment for an occupational therapist, let me tell you. I just sat there behind the wheel of my own car, thinking: 'Yay!'

"For me, working with these patients was a very joyful experience. And I would tell each one: 'Don't get discouraged. You can do this. This could be the beginning of a whole new life for you!'"

"For me, working with these patients was a very joyful experience."
- Joseph Wanchik

Take a Closer Look

Researchers zeroing in on "artificial vision"

Drop by Dr. Raymond Iezzi's busy "artificial vision" lab at the Kresge Eye Institute on a typical weekday afternoon, and the odds are high that you'll find this extraordinary researcher in the middle of a mind-bending project designed to help blind patients see again.

Dr. Iezzi, a New York Medical College-trained physician with a world-class reputation as a cutting-edge explorer of the "physics of human vision," has spent the past decade working to understand how the eye sends millions of "packets of information" to the brain each second in order to trigger the staggeringly complex phenomenon we call "eyesight."

Dr. Iezzi's amazing, long-term goal: To restore vision in blind patients and to prevent the onset of blindness.

His strategy is to explore ways in which "electrode implants" can stimulate the retina, the nerve center where vision begins, in order to restore vision to the blind. By sending tiny amounts of electrical current into the neurons (brain cells) that produce vision, the DMC researcher is better able to understand exactly how the "camera" of the eye transmits similar bursts of electrical energy along the optic nerve for processing by the hard-working brain.

Amazing stuff? You bet. According to Kresge Eye Institute Director Dr. Gary W. Abrams, the day is approaching when computer-based "visualization tools" will begin to replace damaged or non-functioning components of the eye, such as the all-important retina, which registers patterns of light and shadow and then transmits them to the optic nerve for dissemination throughout the brain.

"I don't think we'll reach the point anytime soon where we've got the $6 million man walking around with an artificial eye that sees better than normal," says Dr. Abrams, referring to a popular TV series of the past. "Still, there's no doubt that researchers like our Dr. Iezzi are getting closer every day to giving artificial vision to some blind people.

"But the quest for artificial vision is only one of a dozen different research initiatives now under way at Kresge," adds Dr. Abrams, whose own research into new techniques for

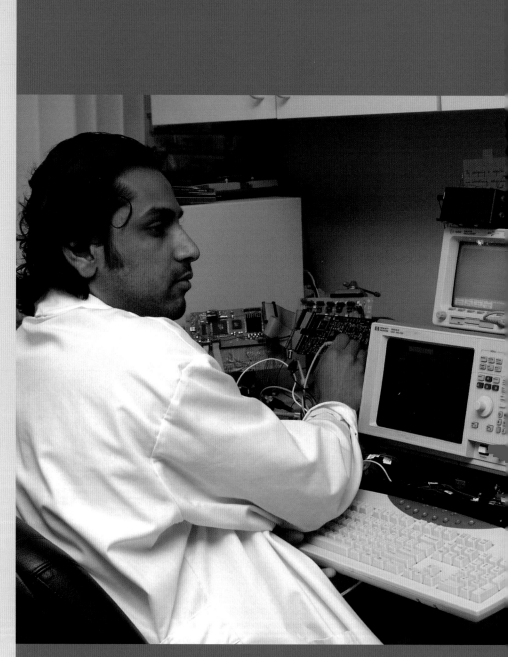

Research at Kresge Eye Institute explores ways "electrode implants" can stimulate the visual cortex.

improving retinal surgery has been widely published in recent years.

"I think the most exciting thing about our research program at Kresge is the way it cuts across so many different specialties in order to bring together the very latest findings from both 'clinical' and 'basic' science. Right now, we've got several different teams of researchers working on cutting-edge issues that range from discovery of the basic mechanisms that cause diabetic eye disease and identifying possible new treatments to refining 'neural protective agents,' a family of specially engineered biochemicals designed to prevent vision-linked brain cells and cells in the retina from deteriorating rapidly as a result of eye-related disorders such as glaucoma, age-related macular degeneration and stroke."

Founded in 1948, the Kresge Eye Institute today treats more than 90,000 patients suffering from eye disorders each year while also performing about 4,000 eye surgeries. Led by a staff of more than 30 M.D. and Ph.D. ophthalmology professionals who also teach at the Wayne State University School of Medicine, Kresge has, in recent years, established an international reputation as a center for both clinical care and research. Among the most exciting of the research initiatives

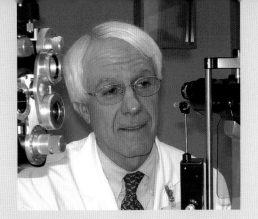

"There's no doubt that researchers are getting closer every day to creating the world's first truly artificial pair of eyes."

- Gary W. Abrams, M.D.

now under way there are these:

• A series of ongoing clinical trials, directed by Kresge researcher Dr. Dean Eliott, aimed at testing new surgical and pharmacological therapies for such chronic ailments as diabetic retinopathy, complex retinal detachment, macular degeneration and pediatric retinal disease.

• A unique array of studies in which Kresge investigator and Wayne State University Ophthalmology Professor Dr. Robert N. Frank is seeking to find new therapies for medical diseases of the retina. As the editor-in-chief of the influential journal *Investigative Ophthalmology and Visual Science*, Dr. Frank is a nationally

renowned expert on both diabetic retinopathy and age-related macular degeneration.

• An ongoing evaluation of the latest generation of "low-vision" tools for patients who are approaching legal blindness, directed by Dr. Iezzi, the scientific director of Kresge's high-tech Ligon Research Center of Vision. With Drs. Nicolas Cottaris and Sylvia Elfar, Dr. Iezzi also conducts research on all aspects of "visual prosthesis" design, including surgical implantation and electrophysiological testing, which is aimed at enhancing the brain's ability to receive and process visual data from the human retina. Such enhancements could one day greatly improve the visual capability of patients affected by retinitis pigmentosa, macular degeneration or other retinal degenerative diseases.

• Improvement in how rapidly the cornea of the eye heals following injury. Dr. Gabriel Sosne is the leading researcher in the country studying the effect of a tissue-derived protein, Thymosin Beta 4 (TB4) on corneal wound healing. Dr. Sosne has demonstrated the ability of TB4 to promote healing of corneal injuries from scratches to severe chemical injuries. Dr. Sosne will lead clinical trials to determine if an eye drop with TB4 will safely and successfully treat corneal injuries in diabetic patients following extensive eye surgery. These studies may lead to a new product to treat eye injuries. Another KEI researcher, Dr. Fu-Shin Yu, the Director of Research at the Institute, is studying the mechanisms of corneal inflammation in order to develop new methods to prevent and treat corneal inflammation and infection.

• Dr. Renu Kowluru is evaluating how oxidative stress (tissue damage due to oxygen-induced substances) damages the blood vessels of the retina in diabetic retinopathy. Dr. Kowluru has shown that prevention of oxidative stress will prevent diabetic retinopathy.

Ask Kresge director Gary Abrams to pull out his crystal ball and speculate about the dramatic breakthroughs that are now taking place in the world of eyecare research, and he won't hesitate with his answer. "I think it's a very exciting time to be an ophthalmologist," says the retinal specialist, "because we are now seeing such a wide array of hopeful advances throughout our field.

"Example: If you look at the new work that's been done — some of it right here at Kresge — in 'teaching' the bipolar cells and the ganglion cells of the retina to take over for damaged photo-receptors in the retina and then send 'light-signals' to the brain, you suddenly realize that this kind of new therapy is going to revolutionize the way we treat patients with such problems as retinitis pigmentosa.

"As a researcher, myself, I find it thrilling to know that we're on the road to preventing — and even reversing — blindness for millions of people all around the globe during the next couple of decades."

Abrams concludes, "What more could a researcher or an administrator hope for than to make an impact like that?"

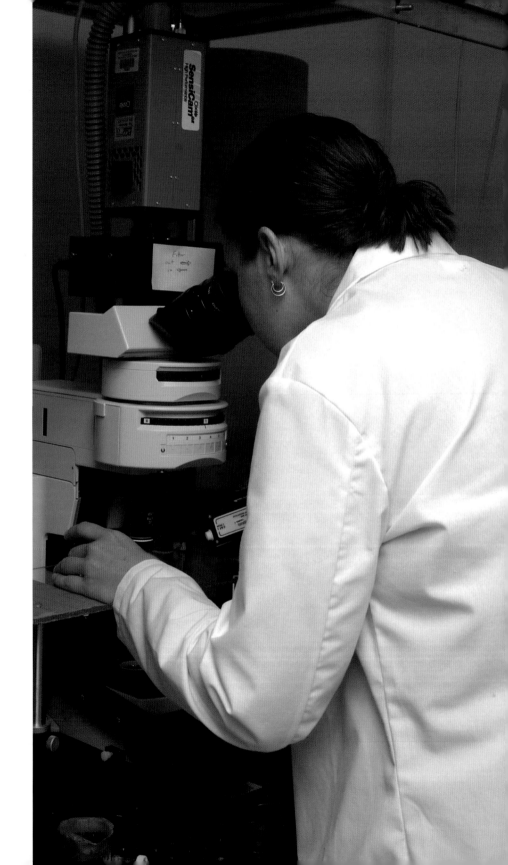

Surgeons rescue child from total blindness

The patient was only eight years old. And he was about to experience a terrible tragedy.

Unless the surgeons at the DMC's Kresge Eye Institute could quickly repair the severely damaged retinas in both his eyes, this unfortunate third-grader would spend the rest of his life in total blindness.

Recalling this "supremely challenging" case of about 15 years ago, Kresge director and veteran eye surgeon Dr. Gary W. Abrams, says the outcome seemed "very much in doubt" at first because it involved a series of highly complex and difficult surgical procedures.

"I remember that case quite vividly," says Dr. Abrams today, "since it eventually required one of the most complicated retinal repair procedures I've ever participated in.

"For starters, this little boy was already blind in one eye, due to a detached retina. At the same time, he also had a huge 'retinal tear' in the other eye. Our assignment was to go in and try to fix the torn retina. But that's a lot easier said than done because, when you're operating on retinal tissue,

the thickness of the material is usually less than one millimeter.

"And when you cut into the retina, the tolerances become even closer. In some areas of the tissue, you're working on layers only microns thick. So we faced an extremely delicate operation. But if this kid was ever going to see again, we had to fix that tear quickly."

And the outcome?

"In that particular case, the outcome was terrific!" says Dr. Abrams. "We got the tissue repaired, and it healed up very nicely. We also reattached the retina in the *other* eye and the young man eventually wound up with very good 20-25 vision as a result.

"As a matter of fact, he recently graduated from college. We keep in touch, and he's doing very well."

And the doctor's reaction?

"What can I say?" booms the enthusiastic Dr. Abrams. "Our surgeons operate on 4,000 patients each year, and when you get a result that saves a child from blindness, you really feel as if your time has been well spent."

Beginning in 1868

The "creative partnership"
brings world-class medical care
to one million patients each year

May 14, 1868

It began quietly enough — on a mild spring afternoon
only a few years after the conclusion of the Civil War —
when a young medical doctor named Ted McGraw
decided to call a meeting of physicians at the brand-new
Harper Hospital in Detroit.

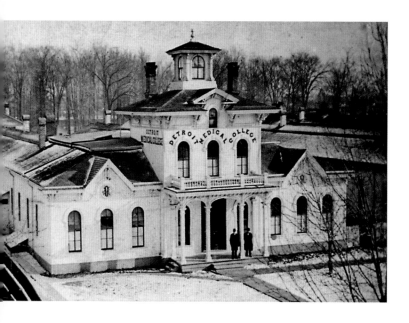

Founded in 1868, the Wayne State University School of Medicine, with more than 1,000 medical students, is now the largest single-campus medical school in the nation. The school offers Master's degree, Ph.D. and M.D. programs in 14 areas of basic science. Today, 60 percent of Michigan physicians receive training at WSU.

As the doctors filed into the tiny auditorium on the second floor of Harper that day, they did not suspect that they were about to participate in a historic moment: the launching of what would someday become the largest single-campus medical school in the United States.

But Dr. McGraw was a man on a mission that day, and he didn't waste any words.

"Good afternoon, gentlemen," he told the small gathering of physicians, most of whom had recently returned from battlefield service with the Union Army, "and thank you for attending this planning session. Today, I want to share with you the prospectus for the new Detroit Medical College, as follows . . ."

A moment later, Dr. McGraw began reading to the assembled physicians a brief report that would soon be filed with the Harper Board of Trustees:

A part of the central portion of the building will be used for a lecture room, semicircular in shape and provided with seats on an inclined plane for about 250 students. Near the main entrance will be a vestibule with a staircase on each side up to the top of the amphitheater, and the dissecting room and laboratory will be in the rear of the lecture room.

By early November of that same year, the first classes had begun at this early ancestor of today's Wayne State University of School of Medicine where some of the world's most promising medical research now takes place daily, and where more than 1,000 medical students now learn the art and science of healing during each semester.

Originally established as the Detroit Medical College and housed during its early years in the original Harper Hospital, the Wayne State University School of Medicine, with more than 1,000 medical students, is now the largest single-campus medical school in the nation. The school offers Master's degree, Ph.D. and M.D. programs in 14 areas of basic science to about 400 students each year.

Wayne State awarded $125 million for research in infant mortality

True or False: Hutzel Women's Hospital — in partnership with the Wayne State University School of Medicine — these days receives more federal research dollars for the study of infant mortality and premature birth than any other teaching hospital in America.

If you answered "True," go immediately to the head of the class where you'll find DMC President and CEO Michael Duggan enthusiastically describing Hutzel's ongoing $125 million, federally sponsored program in neonatal health research.

"Hutzel Women's Hospital has achieved many breakthroughs over the years," says the DMC CEO, "but none was more important than the decision by the National Institutes of Health to establish the nation's only hospital-based perinatology research program right here at Michigan's first and only hospital for women.

"That 10-year research initiative, now being conducted by the NIH's Perinatology Research Branch (PRB) at Hutzel and Wayne State University, offers the promise of some truly exciting breakthroughs in the prevention of premature birth and the reduction of infant mortality rates. Of course, the $125 million federal contract has also begun to pump some welcome resources into the economy of Detroit's midtown and surrounding areas as researchers, medical professionals and related service workers all participate in the research now unfolding daily."

As CEO Duggan is quick to point out, the Perinatology Research Branch is one of only a few NIH intramural branches located outside its main campus in Maryland, and it represents a unique partnership between the NIH and an academic medical center.

At the 134-year-old Hutzel Women's Hospital, meanwhile, they'll tell you that the arrival of the PRB is only the latest in a long series of medical breatkthroughs for this unique medical institution. "Generations of Detroit women have looked to Hutzel Women's Hospital to provide them with outstanding care," says Julia Darlow, nationally known attorney and former chair of the Hutzel Board of Trustees. "Since the day it was founded, Hutzel has provided a leadership role in medical research aimed at improving women's lives."

Founded "by women for women" in 1868, Hutzel is today nationally recognized as a research leader in high-risk obstetrics, infertility, reproductive genetics, gynecology and neonatology.

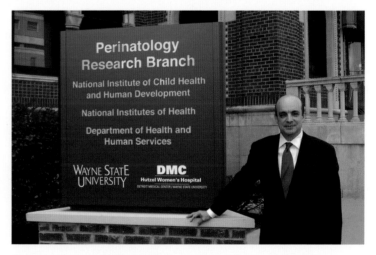

Roberto Romero, M.D.; Chief, Perinatology Research Branch Intramural Division; National Institute of Child Health and Human Development; National Institutes of Health; Department of Health and Human Services

New gamma knife helps to save patient with brain cancer

Roy Gooch says he'll never forget the moment seven years ago when a Detroit neurosurgeon told him he had a brain tumor that might prove fatal.

"I was scared, all right, but not for myself," says the 34-year-old businessman and resident of Kalamazoo. "My two kids were just babies back then, and my cancer diagnosis left me wondering if they'd have to grow up without a father.

"My wife [Tricia] and I sat down and talked it over. We decided that we weren't going to sit around waiting for matters to take their course. We decided to fight back. And we were very fortunate because we soon learned that I might be a candidate for the Gamma Knife."

The break that may have saved Roy Gooch's life came when an old college friend, an RN working in Detroit, told him about a brand-new cancer-fighting weapon that had just gone online at the Detroit Medical Center's Harper University Hospital.

That weapon was a high-tech "radiotherapy" device, originally developed in Sweden, which can focus 201 different gamma rays on a single, millimeter-wide segment of brain tissue. Known medically as the Gamma Knife, this computer-driven, high-tech device can apply enormous radio energy to a tiny surface in order to wipe out cancer cells while avoiding healthy tissue located nearby.

The story of how Roy Gooch's doctors used this extraordinary tool to completely eliminate his brain-stem carcinoma in 1997 has provided a hopeful note for cancer patients all across the Midwest in recent years, according to medical researchers.

Precise, Non-invasive and Low-risk

The Gooch medical drama began in the fall of 1997 when Roy checked into the DMC in order to receive a biopsy of a suspicious growth that had been discovered during a post-automobile-accident brain scan in Kalamazoo.

The biopsy confirmed the presence of a small cancer lesion on his brain stem, a key area of the brain that controls such vital bodily functions as eye movement and sleeping.

For Roy Gooch, whose family runs a busy printing-supply store in Kalamazoo, the bad news was that most cancers in this sensitive

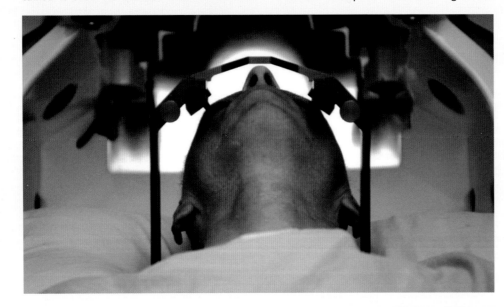

The gamma knife is precise, non-invasive and low risk, but it can also be more effective.

area cannot be operated on by traditional methods. The risk of a disabling brain injury is simply too great.

But there was also some good news — the fact that his lesion was small enough and undeveloped enough to be vulnerable to the intense beams of radiation that can be directed by the Gamma Knife surgical device. At that time, the DMC operated the only Gamma Knife radiotherapy system in the entire state of Michigan.

After discussing Roy's case thoroughly with a colleague in Radiation Oncology, Dr. Kenneth Levin, a veteran DMC physician specially trained in radiotherapy, recommended the Gamma Knife for his Kalamazoo patient.

Why? According to Dr. Levin's careful analysis, the benefits that could be expected from this form of therapy far outweighed the risks. Among the advantages he noted were these:

• The Gamma Knife could be expected to apply a huge dose of cancer-killing radiation directly to the tumor, accurate to one or two millimeters, while leaving other essential brain tissue unaffected.

• The patient would experience very little discomfort, and the absence of an incision would eliminate the risks of hemorrhage and infection.

• Because the surgery was non-invasive, Roy's hospital stay could be limited to a single night.

It didn't take the Gooches long to reach their decision after listening to the neurosurgeon's assessment of risks and benefits. On December 20, 1997, he checked back into the DMC and underwent a painless, 12-minute procedure in which the 201 gamma rays were programmed by a specialized computer to attack the lesion that threatened his life.

"The Gamma Knife procedure went very well that day," recalls Dr. Levin, who has conducted hundreds of similar treatments with it during recent years. "Because the computer technology and the imaging system are so precise and easy to operate, I was able to direct the movement of the [radiation] beams with great precision.

"We finished the entire procedure in about 12 minutes, and the patient said he experienced very little discomfort. I felt pretty confident when we were finished that we had taken care of the problem. Seven years later, an MRI confirmed that there was no cancer present.

"Mr. Gooch tells me that he's in very good health these days, and that's the kind of outcome I really like."

Ask Roy Gooch to describe what it felt like to go under the Gamma Knife, and he'll surprise you by chuckling out loud. "Really, I felt no sensation at all," says the former hard-charging forward for the Rochester (Mich.) Adams High School Highlanders basketball team. "As I told Tricia later, the toughest part of the entire operation was when they put that steel ring [frame] around my head to keep it still while the gamma rays did their work."

Years after receiving the medical diagnosis that changed their lives, Roy and Tricia Gooch say they're "eager to spread the word" about the importance of self-education for cancer patients. "We feel very blessed and very lucky to have come through the experience in such a positive way," says Tricia. "I think we were very fortunate to have learned about the Gamma Knife procedure, and I would urge cancer patients to learn all they can about such tools."

For his part, Roy says he is also grateful for the fact that "my illness actually brought our family closer together." Having survived the onslaught of cancer for years now, he says he and Tricia have learned "to enjoy every single moment we have together." Accompanied by their new puppy, the floppy-eared "Wyatt," the Gooch family spends "almost every weekend" on the beach at South Haven or frolicking with a Frisbee in their own Kalamazoo backyard.

At the DMC, meanwhile, Gamma Knife practitioner Dr. Levin says he was also quite pleased by the results. "Mr. Gooch has done quite well since his treatment here, and that's very encouraging for all of us. Our goal is to make this powerful technology available to cancer patients everywhere so that they can take maximum advantage of it."

Today's school of medicine

Teaching students the art and science of medicine is only part of the daily challenge. From the day it opened more than 135 years ago, Detroit's only medical school has also dedicated itself to cutting-edge research. After decades of robust scientific inquiry into medical topics that range from premature birth and neonatal intensive care to hypertension and diabetes in urban populations, it's no surprise to discover that the Wayne State School of Medicine now ranks 22nd in total research expenditures among U.S. med schools — with a research portfolio of more than $135 million annually, according to the National Science Foundation. Among the key areas of research today — as reported in major medical and scientific journals all across the country — are investigations into the causes and treatment of cancer, women's and children's health, neuroscience and population studies.

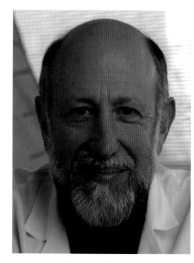

Robert R. Frank, M.D.

Another major area of WSU study through the years has been research into reproductive health. Today, Wayne State's Department of Obstetrics and Gynecology ranks first in the country in total research funding from the National Institutes of Health. And the department also provides a home to the NIH Perinatology Research Branch, which is dedicated to improving the quality of maternal-fetal health nationwide. That same department has been a major pioneer in several innovative therapies, including fetal surgery to treat birth defects in the womb, the first-ever successful in-utero bone-marrow transplant, and Michigan's first in-vitro fertilization program.

Today, the WSU School of Medicine is affiliated with the hospitals in the Detroit Medical Center, including the Children's Hospital of Michigan, the Rehabilitation Institute of Michigan, Hutzel Women's Hospital, Detroit Receiving Hospital, Harper University Hospital, Huron Valley-Sinai Hospital, Sinai-Grace Hospital and the Michigan Orthopaedic Specialty Hospital.

The school also offers a major program of emphasis in the neurosciences, including neurology, neurotrauma, neuromuscular and degenerative diseases, vision sciences, neurobehavioral sciences and neuro-imaging. Another highly innovative WSU program can be found at the Rehabilitation Institute of Michigan's Center for Spinal Cord Injury Recovery.

Describing these and other cutting-edge research programs, WSU School of Medicine Dean Robert R. Frank, M.D., says he's "more excited than ever about the prospects for groundbreaking research" at the medical school, because of the "unique partnership" between one of the nation's most highly rated training programs for new physicians and the urban hospitals where they practice their skills daily.

"There's no doubt that the model of the 'teaching hospital' has been shown to provide the most effective — and the most economical — system for maintaining high-quality medical care in the urban setting," says the enthusiastic Dr. Frank. "These days, I'm convinced as never before that the 'teaching hospital' continues to be one of the most effective and financially feasible public health institutions now serving the American public."

As the only medical school in Detroit, Dr. Frank notes, Wayne State has a historical mission to promote public health in the city. To that end, the school recently received a $6 million NIH grant to create the Center for Urban & African-American Health, an initiative that will seek new ways to correct health care disparities by finding new therapeutic approaches to chronic diseases in this population, such as obesity, cardiovascular disease and cancer.

Perhaps the greatest contribution to the community by the school is its treatment of patients who are under-insured or who lack insurance altogether. Along with the DMC, Wayne State physicians provide an average of $150 million in uncompensated medical care each year.

In addition, the Wayne State University School of Medicine is nationally recognized for its biomedical research. Areas of particular excellence within the School of Medicine include the neuorosciences and advanced imaging, women's and children's health, cancer, and urban and African-American health studies. Strong programmatic emphasis is also placed on the integration of the basic and clinical sciences through interdisciplinary research, which has led to the creation of several university institutes and centers.

As Dr. Frank likes to point out whenever possible, Wayne State School of Medicine faculty hold many key positions in Detroit Medical Center hospitals. The DMC today offers a combined total of more than 2,400 licensed beds, making it one of the largest medical centers in the country. Each year, DMC hospitals log more than 87,000 admission and 900,000 outpatient visits. And more than 2,400 physicians and fellows provide this care along with more than 1,000 medical students and about 14,000 full-time employees.

During more than a century of partnership, this "creative partnership" between the public university and the urban hospitals has continued to provide outstanding medical care for Detroit residents, which, come to think of it, is exactly what Dr. Ted McGraw had in mind on that warm spring day in 1868 when the first chapter in the saga of the "Detroit Medical College" got its start.

"The model of the 'teaching hospital' has been shown to provide the most effective and the most economical system for maintaining high-quality medical care in the urban setting."

- Robert R. Frank, M.D.

Academic medical center leads the way to the latest in technological breakthroughs

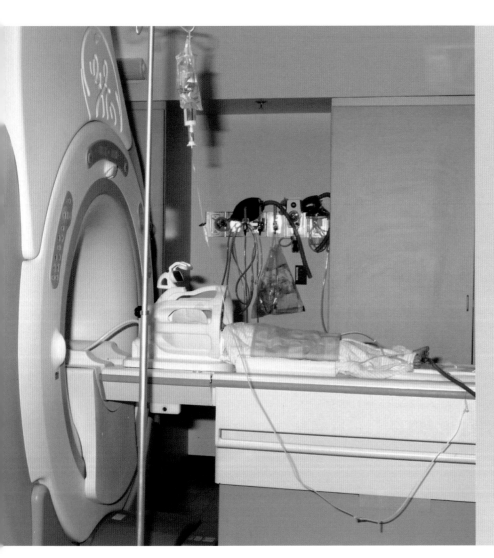

Detroit's home to one of the nation's only 3T MR with a short bore

As MR technology becomes intricate in diagnosing sports-related injures, vascular and cardiovascular needs and other neuro-imaging areas, Children's Hospital of Michigan is one of the first pediatric centers to add a 3T MR, short bore. MR is imaging quickly displacing CT and nuclear medicine in many areas. 3T refers to the strength of the magnet. In addition, the length of the new scanner opening for the patient is much shorter. It is perfect for children, helping to prevent claustrophobia and reducing the need for sedation in children.

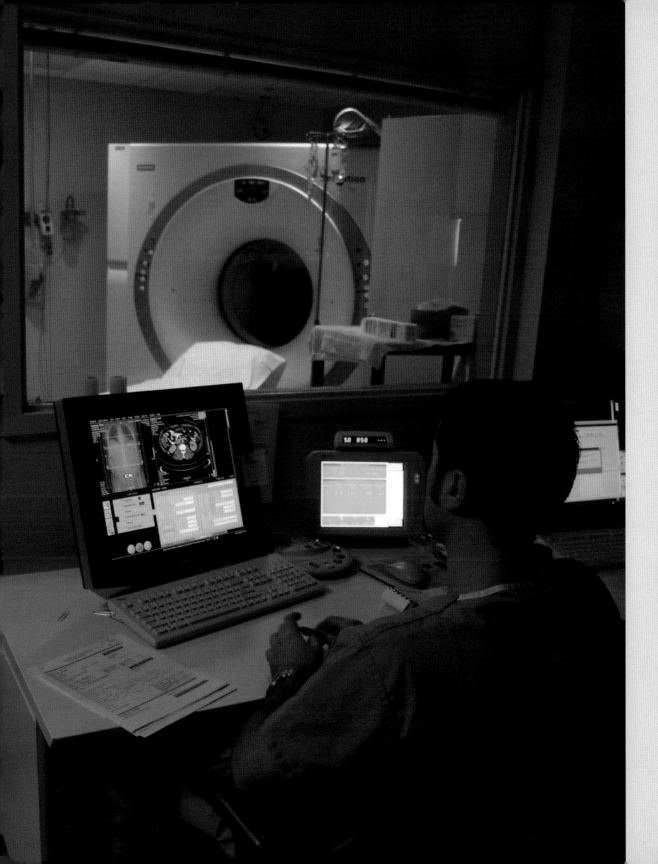

64-Slice Computed Tomography (CT) scanner offers fast, painless exams to catch disease early

Harper University Hospital was one of the first in Michigan to use 64-slice computed tomography (CT) scans to detect disease earlier than ever before. The 64-CT Slice is able to non-invasively capture thousands of three-dimensional, high-resolution images in seconds with fewer complicaions for the patient. This latest technology enables physicians to more quickly and accurately visualize abnormalities than any other non-invasive CT testing available, drastically improving patient outcomes in the areas of cardiology, vascular surgery, neurology and surgery.

Specialists remove a brain tumor during scalpel-free, minimally invasive surgery

August, 2003. It was late afternoon on the Detroit River and 27-year-old rowing competitor Domenic DeCaria had just returned from a lengthy practice session to his Wyandotte boat slip. As he stepped from his rowing scull to the wet pine planks of the dock, he was looking forward to a cold brew at a nearby pub.

But moments later, disaster struck.

Domenic's right foot skidded on a patch of algae and he plunged headfirst. A moment later — **POW!** — his head struck the side of the dock, knocking him unconscious. Horrified, several other members of the Wyandotte Boat Club (along with his terrified mother, who'd come to the dock to pick him up that day) quickly pulled the youthful DeCaria from the water and did their best to revive him. Although the Trenton rower was soon awake, he remained "dizzy and delirious." Increasingly concerned, his fretful mother insisted that he visit a local community hospital for a CT scan that would determine whether or not he'd received a significant brain injury.

Although the accident seemed unlucky at first, Domenic eventually realized that his mishap on the water was actually a stroke of good fortune. He came to that conclusion after the CT scan at the local hospital revealed that he had a pituitary tumor growing inside his skull with a potential to expand and cause blindness.

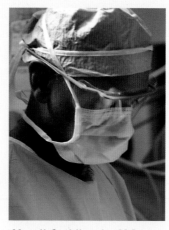

Murali Guthikonda, M.D.

"At first, I was freaked out by the results of the CT scan," says Domenic today. "But then I realized that the accident had been a good thing because a pituitary tumor may not cause any symptoms until it gets very large and more difficult to treat. Because of that boating accident, I received an early warning about the cancer in my brain, and I was able to get treatment in a hurry."

That treatment began in earnest when the young man checked into a surgical unit at Harper University Hospital where a skilled neurosurgeon who specializes in treating brain and pituitary tumors was soon able to help him. After ordering an MRI and studying the results in careful detail, the highly regarded specialist — Harper Chief of Neurosurgery Murali Guthikonda, M.D. — recommended that the patient undergo an innovative, high-tech form of brain surgery that doesn't require an incision.

Domenic and his family quickly agreed to this treatment plan, and in October 2003 the "minimally invasive" procedure took place in an operating room at Harper.

In order to remove the cancer, the veteran DMC surgeon inserted a tiny scope through the patient's nasal passage and sinus cavity. Once inside the affected area of the brain, the scope becomes a scalpel, and Dr. Guthikonda used it to remove every last trace of the hidden carcinoma.

The results were impressive, to say the least. Because the tumor had grown on only one side of the pituitary gland, the surgeon was able to remove it completely, while leaving enough gland to provide necessary hormones. Since then, Domenic has been cancer-free and his vision has not been affected at all by the surgery. Nor is the patient required to take medications daily for the rest of his life, which would have been the case if his pituitary gland had been removed.

After nearly two decades as a brain surgeon, Dr. Guthikonda says that "knowing how to plan every detail of surgery well in advance is the key to being effective in the operating room. In a certain sense, brain surgery is a little bit like chess; you have to have a clear, thought-out plan that will achieve the final outcome you want.

"As you might expect, I spend many hours reviewing CT scans and lab tests aimed at defining the patient's health problem as accurately as possible. Then I spend more hours mapping out a plan of attack in the operating room. The plan can get quite complicated at times because you have to have a response ready for every single thing that could happen during brain surgery.

"But over the years, I've learned that if you plan well, things will usually go well in that operating room."

Like Domenic DeCaria, who has long since returned to the rowing competition he loves, the U.S. National Cancer Institute in recent years has recognized the excellence of cancer treatment and clinical research at the DMC by certifying the programs as one of only 39 NCI-sanctioned "National Cancer Centers" in the United States.

Says a grateful Domenic, more than two years after the surgery left him cancer-free, "I feel great today. I'm in better shape than ever, and I'm out there on the water and rowing hard again. The care I received at the DMC was outstanding and, because it was minimally invasive, I went home after only three days in the hospital. Nor did I experience any significant discomfort except for the fact that I wasn't allowed to sneeze for a solid month.

"I also grew closer to my mom during this experience, which was a terrific side benefit. She was at my bedside day and night, and she never stopped trying to help me. I learned all over again that she's the best friend I have in the world, and I'm extremely grateful to her for that.

"I'm also grateful to the doctors and nurses at the DMC for making my stay there so comfortable. The surgery was swift, painless and without significant side effects, and it eliminated the tumor completely, so I could get on with my life!"

"The surgery was swift, painless and without significant side effects, and it eliminated the tumor completely, so I could get on with my life!"

- Domenic DeCaria

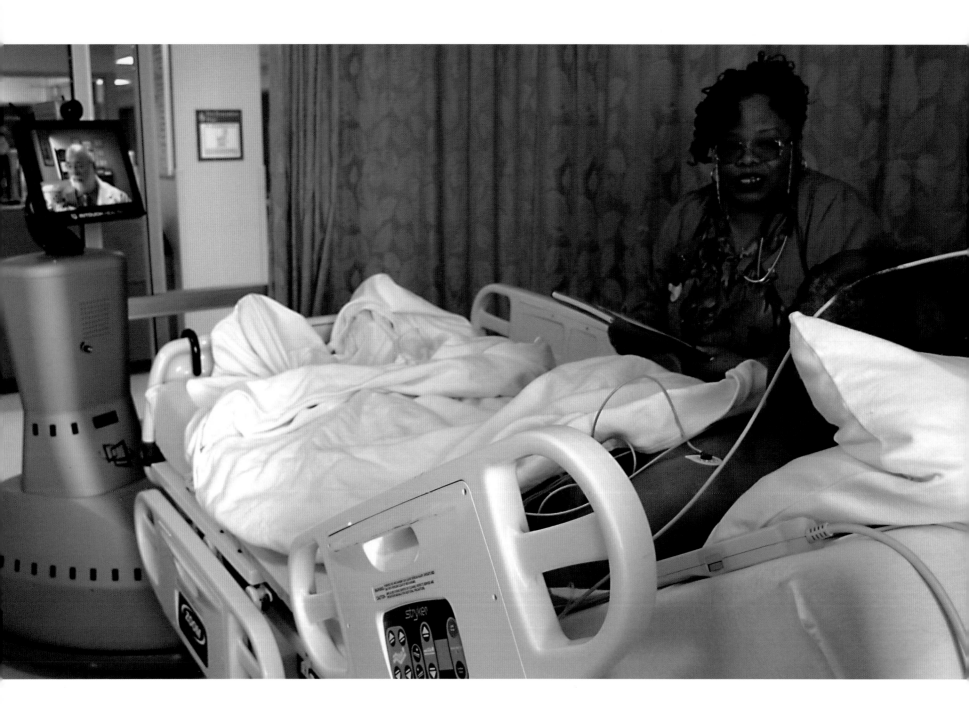

R2D2? No, it's Metro Detroit's fleet of robo docs

It's Monday morning at Harper University Hospital, and Dr. Joseph Bander has decided he needs to make a bedside visit to a patient on a distant ward.

But there's a problem.

Because the IC Unit at Harper is crowded with patients, Dr. Bander must remain at his office. He's in charge of the unit right now, and he certainly can't take off on a lengthy trek to the ward where a struggling patient needs to be evaluated.

Anybody got a solution?

You bet! Why not page Dr. Bander's high-tech assistant, a computer-driven, self-propelled, video robot known as "RP-6?"

Can the always-energetic "robot doctor" help make the patient evaluation in the far-off ward?

In a scenario that resembles something out of Star Wars, the busy ICU physician quickly slides behind a computer terminal in his office and grabs the "joystick" that controls the movements of his mobile robot. A moment later, Dr. Bander is guiding the flickering, rubber-wheeled device along a crowded Harper hallway.

At five feet, three inches of height, the "smart robot" bears a remarkable resemblance to R2D2 and several other humanoids of sci-fi fame as it loops around corners, boards elevators and even "looks" for the room number through a specially mounted video camera.

After an Internet-directed journey of several minutes, the robot finds the patient's room and joins a nurse who's changing a bandage on the patient's wound.

Still seated in his own office, Dr. Bander watches the procedure unfold while carefully studying such important medical details as the color of the wound-discharge and the amount of difficulty the patient has breathing. With his own smiling face lighting up RP-6's video screen, Dr. Bander questions the nurse about the patient's condition.

When he wants a closer look, the ICU doc maneuvers the joystick, which pushes the two-mile-an-hour-max robot in closer to bedside. Dr. Bander can now scrutinize such telltale evidence as skin tone, breathing rate and sleeping posture.

A few minutes later, thanks to the help from his robot-assistant, Dr. Bander can make a well-informed decision about treatment. In this case, he decides that the patient doesn't need to be moved to ICU, although he will ask the nurse to keep a close eye on the figure in the bed during the next few hours.

Now Doctors Can Be in "Two Places at Once"

They aren't intended to replace the doctor. To the contrary, their purpose is to make contact between doctor and patient (and the patient's family) much more frequent.

"I was skeptical at first, I have to admit it," says the 55-year-old Dr. Bander. "I'm a hands-on kind of doctor, and it was hard for me to imagine a robot helping me to care for patients. And yet the patients seem to love it. Most of them aren't bothered at all by talking to a video screen. And many of the younger patients, like my own kids, grew up using joysticks and playing computer games, so they feel right at home with this kind of technology."

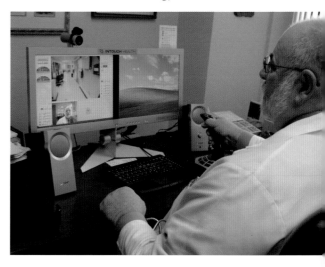

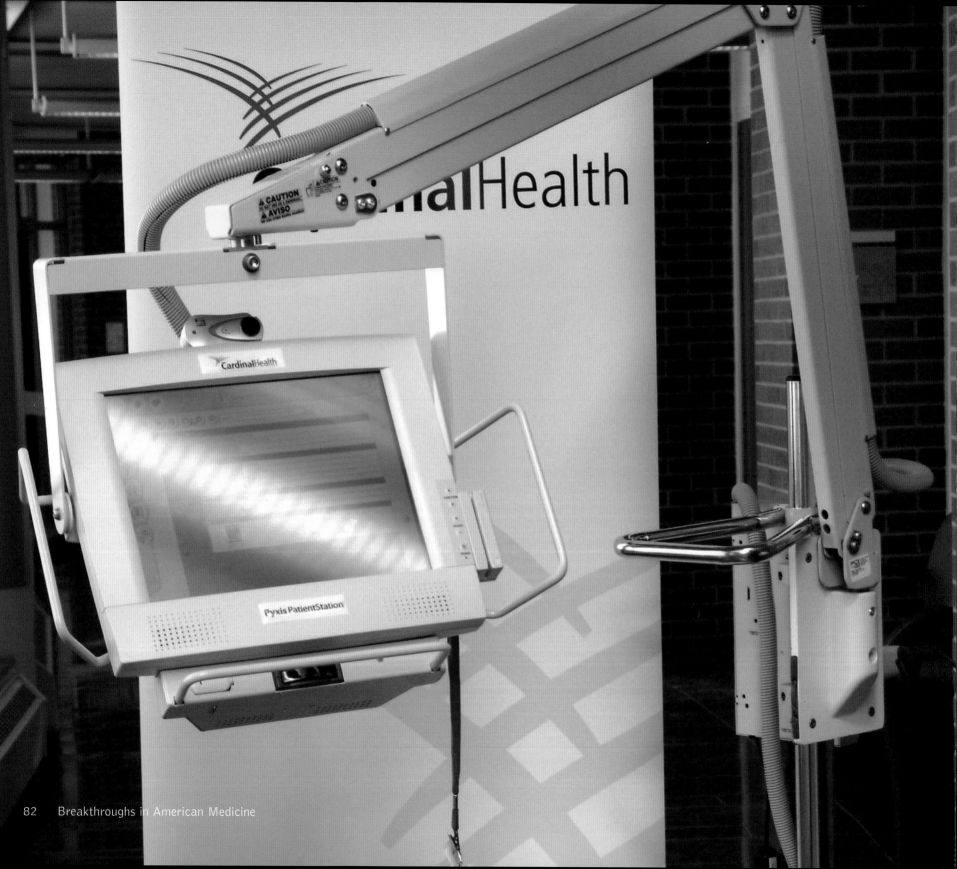

PatientStation: Right time, right place medicine

Take a stroll through one of the wards at the state-of-the-art Huron Valley-Sinai Hospital, and you'll probably be surprised to find many of the patients perched on the sides of their beds while banging away at video games, sending e-mails to friends and even studying their own medical issues on Web sites provided by the hospital staff.

At Huron Valley-Sinai, the first hospital in the United States to install these innovative "PatientStations" next to each and every bed back in 2002, the specially designed computer terminals help to alleviate the boredom that used to be part of every overnight stay at a hospital.

But the nifty devices are also used for an important medical purpose: They allow doctors, nurses and technicians to review lab results, study x-rays, evaluate medical histories and peruse drug charts, never leaving the patient's bedside.

Anchored to a bedside computer terminal with a flat, 15-inch, touch-screen monitor, the "Pyxis PatientStation" gives doctors and nurses instant access to medical literature and medication information worldwide. Best of all, the service (which also includes cable television and movies on demand) is located only a hand-shake-distance from each of the 153 non-emergency beds in the hospital.

The Pyxis system, now being installed in many hospitals around the country, can provide significant assistance to clinicians who say it allows them to spend more time with their patients rather than scooting up and down hallways in search of medical information required for consultations.

Installed in late 2002, the PatientStations have been a hit with patients, more than 60 percent of whom choose to logon to the sleek-looking terminals each day, according to a recent survey. "We've been using these new bedside stations for a couple of years now," says Linda Bell, a Huron Valley-Sinai nurse clinician, "and the results speak for themselves.

"The patients really enjoy the convenience these terminals provide, and they enjoy the chance to watch movies or play video games or check their e-mail. At the same time, these bedside computers really simplify the task of making [medical] rounds each day. I don't think any of us want to go back to racing constantly back and forth along the hallways in order to locate the medical information we need."

Another advantage: Parents who accompany their children to the hospital for overnight stays no longer have to haul TV sets, PlayStations and the like from the house to the car to the hospital room.

Recently endorsed by the American Hospital Association, the Pyxis PatientStation also helps to reduce medical errors by providing clinicians with devices that centrally store and integrate all test results, charts and histories related to each patient's care.

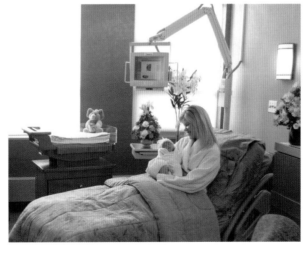

"Our patients tell us all the time how much they like having this kind of convenience at their besides," says Bell. "If you look at patient satisfaction and the clinical advantages, together, it's obvious that the PatientStations are a win-win situation for everyone involved."

In the Beginning . . .
There Were Donors

"We make a living by what we do,
but we make a life by what we give."

-Winston Churchill

It's one of the most dramatic — and yet least known —
stories in the annals of Detroit health care. It's the
story of famed Michigan entrepreneur Peter Karmanos
and how he donated many of the funds required to
build what now ranks as one of the nation's most
accomplished cancer research facilities.

But it's also the story of legendary whiskey entrepreneur Hiram Walker, whose generosity inspired the creation of today's award-winning Children's Hospital of Michigan, and the story of the civic-minded manufacturer William Carls, who spent 20 years helping to raise the funds that built Huron Valley-Sinai Hospital in Oakland County. It is also a look back at the remarkably generous Brasza family whose major gifts helped launch the state-of-the-art Rehabilitation Institute of Michigan's outpatient clinic now bearing their name.

There were thousands of them, philanthropists, physicians of all specialties, big and small, and today, their spirit lives on in the medical facilities — and in the research breakthroughs that their generosity made possible.

While we can't even begin to recognize all the gifts, it is what has been given — big or small — that makes the breakthroughs possible.

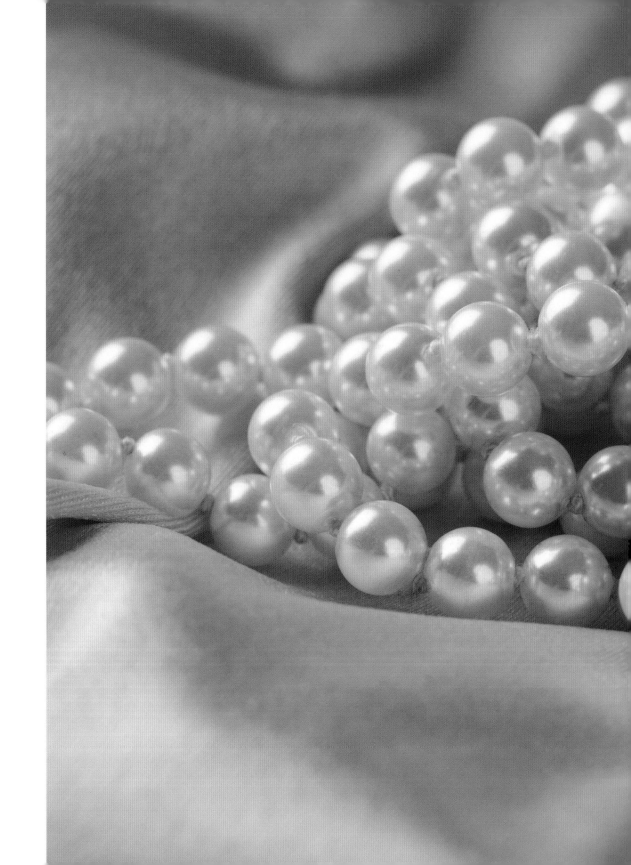

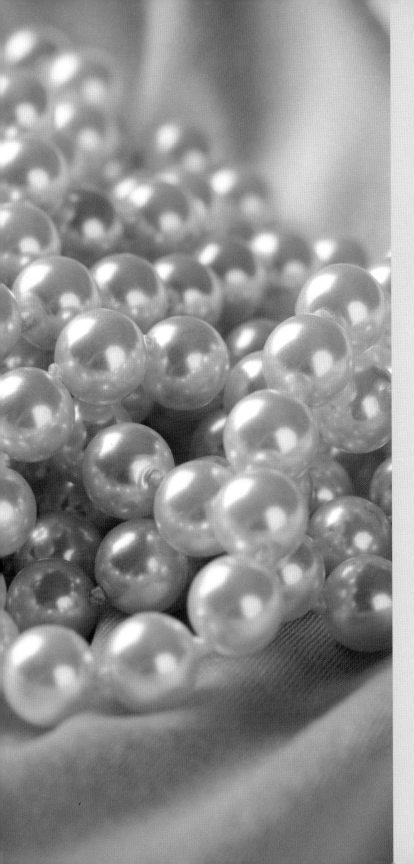

Philanthropist gave beloved spouse "a box for her pearls"

One of the most remarkable philanthropic stories to emerge through the years was surely the dramatic saga of former Ford Motor executive and late United States Senator James Couzens who gave more than $30 million to charity during the 1930s. Those gifts included a $1 million award to Children's Hospital of Michigan, a contribution that still ranks as one of the most significant grants in the history of Michigan philanthropy.

The Couzens contribution to Children's actually got its start as a "birthday request" from the senator's wife. When asked what gift she wanted from her wealthy husband, she pointed out that she "already had everything." All she needed now, she told him, was "a simple box in which to store my precious pearls."

Couzens complied. But when his delighted wife opened the "box," she received an unexpected surprise. Inside, she found a loving note describing how her husband had just donated $1 million to Children's. *My dear*, he reportedly explained in the missive, *your new pearls will be all the children who are eventually treated there.*

The Couzens' gift was only one of the many legendary acts of philanthropy that have helped to support the research, technology and state-of-the-art clinical procedures to be found today at the Detroit Medical Center.

At the dawn of medical care, Harper's gift helped "sick and aged"

If you want to touch the true spirit that guides the Detroit Medical Center and its 14,000 employees throughout the daily struggle to care for patients from all across Michigan, the best place to start is Elmwood Cemetery.

For it is here on a rolling, emerald-green landscape punctuated by majestic oak trees that the original founders of what eventually became the DMC are taking their eternal rest.

To really *feel* their spirit, it's best to drop by 150-year-old Elmwood (the oldest non-religious cemetery in Detroit) on a mild, drowsy, summer afternoon. As for your "guide" on this brief tour, why not choose one of the DMC's most widely admired veteran physicians, the recently retired *gray eminence* of surgery at Harper Hospital, Dr. Agustin Arbulu?

A thoughtful, gentle-voiced man, the longtime cardio-thoracic surgeon and former Chief of Staff (1998-2004) at Harper has done a great deal of historical research on the founding of his hospital, way back in 1859.

"It's no accident that Walter Harper and Nancy Martin wound up here at Elmwood," says the DMC guru with a quiet smile, as we amble toward their resting places at Elmwood, which is located in a pleasant residential neighborhood on Detroit's near east side. Then, waving toward the graceful sculptures and nodding tree branches that dominate the 86-acre burying ground: "Back in the 19th century, most of the city's most respected leaders and philanthropists were buried here. If you look around, you'll find the graves of 11 former U.S. Senators and 28 Detroit Mayors, among many other notables."

He pauses for a moment as we approach a large, rectangular block of granite that marks two closely adjoining gravesites. "There are a lot of famous Michiganders buried at Elmwood," says the surgeon, "but my favorite monument is *that* one, right over there."

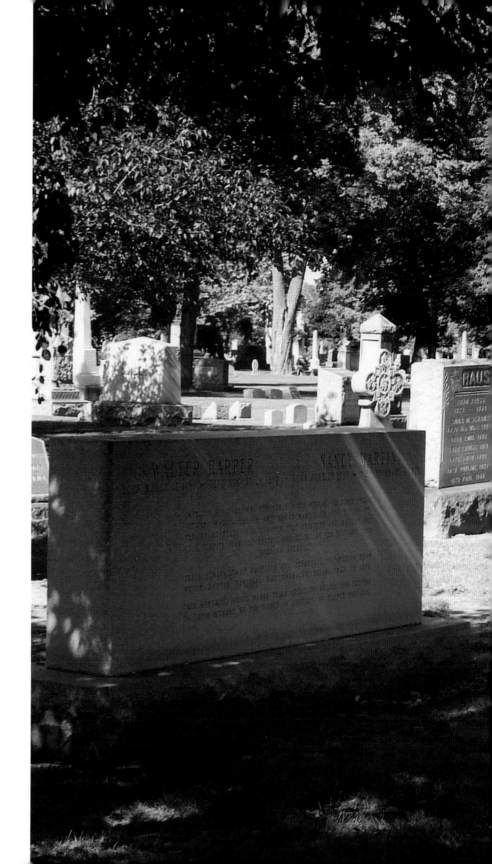

"You know, I spent a lot of years as Chief of Staff at Harper," says Dr. Arbulu after reading the epitaph aloud, "and I've always felt that this memorial perfectly expresses the spirit of our mission at the DMC. Among many other things, we have always been a place where medical care was available to the poor. And I think we have honored that pledge. I think we have welcomed it through the years because it forms the heart of our mission."

That mission began on a cold, blustery evening in February of 1859, when half a dozen of Detroit's leading citizens arrived at the home of a local Presbyterian Minister, the Rev. Dr. George Duffield. Their purpose was simple in concept but would prove complicated in the execution; they were about to formally accept the donation from two wealthy Detroit merchants Walter Harper and Nancy Martin of nearly 1,000 acres of city land that would serve as the headquarters for the city's first full-service hospital dedicated to caring for the poor.

Located in midtown Detroit near the heart of what is today the DMC, the Harper-Martin gift of 864 acres of prime real estate was undoubtedly the single-most important contribution to the hospital group in its entire 150-year history.

In the decades ahead, this huge gift would pave the way not only for Harper University Hospital (soon to be joined in partnership with the Wayne State University School of Medicine), but also for the other Detroit-area medical facilities and clinics that make up the heart of the largest hospital center in Michigan.

Describing the value and the spirit behind this history-making act of philanthropy, the Detroit *Daily Advertiser* would wax especially eloquent:

"It strikes us that the people of Detroit owe it to themselves to give some public expression of the estimation in which they hold the noble act of Nancy Martin in presenting to this city, her beautiful lot on Woodward Avenue. . . . In consideration of this liberal act, can our citizens do less than raise [a matching] amount by subscription, and thus have the whole gift unimpaired for the object for which she designs it? We bravely make the suggestion, and if thought worth anything, it will probably be acted upon. But it seems to us that Detroit can afford to do this much towards the benevolent enterprise which she and Mr. [Walter] Harper have so munificently endowed."

Epitaph

Walter Harper. Born March 17, 1789; died August 28, 1867

Nancy Martin. Born June 25, 1799; died February 9, 1875

Impelled by an abiding concern for the welfare of their fellow citizens, Walter Harper and Nancy Martin in 1859 deeded extensive property holdings for the erection and maintenance of a hospital for the benefit and relief of the sick and aged poor of Detroit. Their benefactions provided the financial foundation upon which Harper Hosptial was formally established in 1863. This monument, which marks their adjoining graves, was erected to their memory by the Board of Trustees of Harper Hospital.

Medical "Art Impresario"
Irene Walt curates largest hospital gallery in the country

If you want to understand Irene Walt's passion for bringing art into public spaces, all you have to do is spend a couple of hours wandering through Detroit Receiving Hospital with her.

Stand in front of the soaring "Giant Steps" sculpture, a 40-foot-high maze of glittering steel tubing that looms like a colossus above a third-floor courtyard, and you'll begin to feel the power of her visionary approach to "enhancing the hospital environment" by transforming it into a vibrant museum for modern art.

Executed by famed Chicago artist Richard Hunt and commissioned back in 1982 as a memorial to former Detroit Mayor Coleman A. Young, "Giant Steps" glides above the once-drab hospital courtyard like an immense, sun-bright falcon caught forever in the moment of taking flight.

For Irene Walt, now 82, the Hunt sculpture at the DMC provides a "marvelous example" of how works of art can "humanize and beautify" public spaces and thus improve the quality of life for visitors, residents and on-site workers alike.

After devoting much of the past 31 years to building what now ranks as one of the world's largest hospital-based art collections, Walt says she greatly enjoys taking visitors on tours of the 900 paintings and sculptures contained in Detroit Receiving's on-site "galleries."

"We raised hundreds of thousands of dollars over the years for art at the hospital," says Irene, "and we also gave many Michigan artists a space in which to display their works. We refurbished dozens of wards with paintings and linen drapes, and as you might imagine, that required a great deal of work from our committee members.

"I can remember times when we worked through the night to mail out more than a thousand fund-raising letters at a time. It was very challenging. Those were the 'infancy days' of putting art into hospitals, starting back in the early 1970s, and those of us who worked on the campaigns felt a great deal of passion and determination on this subject!"

Encouraged by her physician-husband — Alexander J. Walt, who served for 23 years as Chief of Surgery at the Wayne State University School of Medicine before his death in 1996 — the highly regarded consultant Irene Walt first became interested in enhancing public spaces with art way back in 1968. Dr. Walt came home from work one day and challenged her with a special request: "Why don't you come down to Detroit Receiving Hospital and see if you can decorate our eight offices there? The place looks so drab and dull that it's become rather depressing! The residents needed a better place to do their work."

Irene didn't hesitate. Within a few weeks (and after "borrowing half a dozen different art works from my neighbors, permanently!"), she had transformed Receiving's sterile-looking office environment into a mini-art gallery.

What followed was an unprecedented public campaign in which Mrs. Walt convinced a few select Michigan business

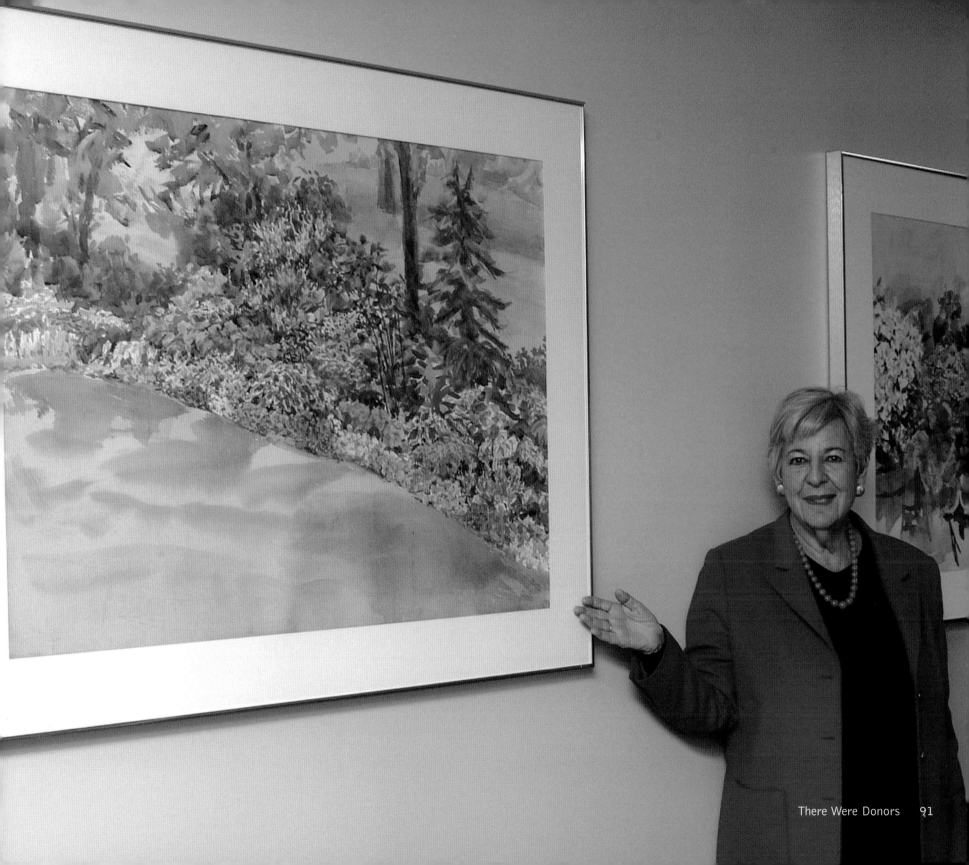

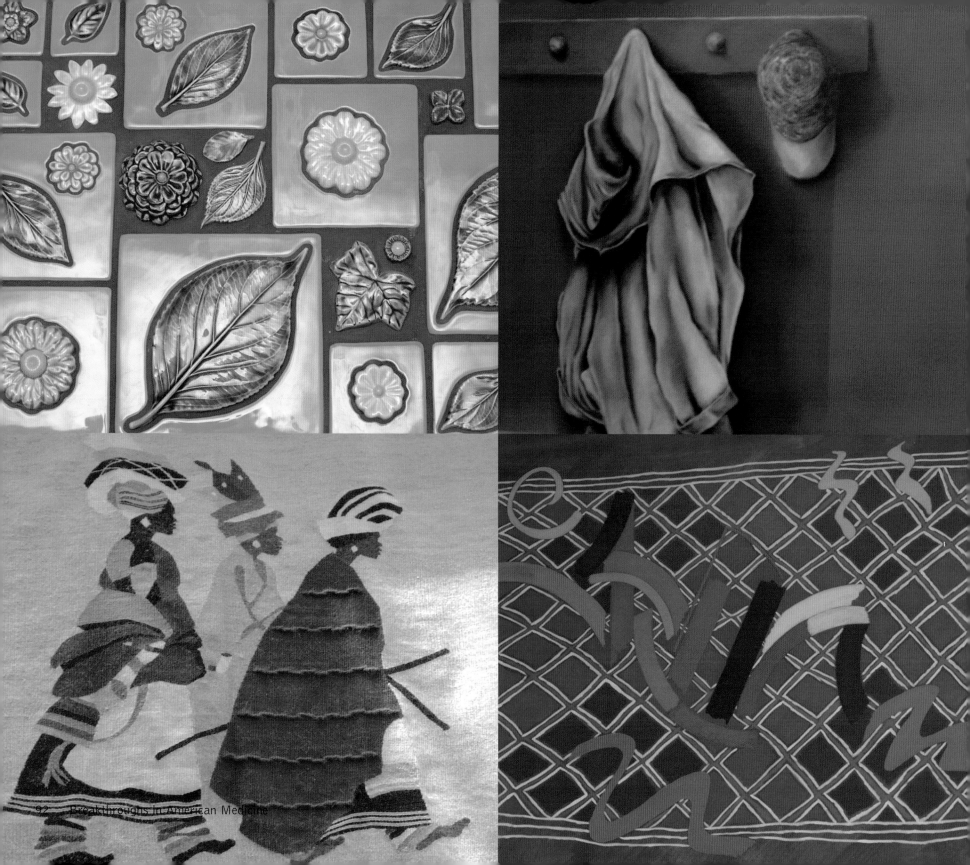

leaders and artists alike to donate time, money and works of art. "Those years were exciting and challenging," she says. "Money was tight, and it wasn't easy. But I found that I often got good results whenever I told a Michigan business executive, 'Nothing is too good for our patients and our staff.'"

Today, the results speak for themselves. Drop by Detroit Receiving Hospital or the nearby University Health Center, and you'll find yourself strolling through an astonishing series of mini-galleries with more than 900 sculptures, paintings, works on paper, textiles and crafts. In recent years, the collection has expanded to include many examples of African beadwork, along with elegant tapestries from the U.S., Africa and Colombia. Other artistic attractions include two major Pewabic tile works, Jeff Guido's large ceramic flower tiles and a series of giant-sized photographic murals located in the lighting above the beds of the Emergency Department. In addition, the new Emergency entrance features a major Glen Michaels Installation and a Charles McGee Aluminum Sculpture.

As the DMC art collection gained fame over the years, Irene Walt found her special skills were in demand on the local scene. In recent years, for example, she led a successful campaign to place more than $2.5 million worth of tile murals, mosaics, neon lighting, paintings and bronze sculptures in the 13 "People Mover" stations that now form the heart of Detroit's public transportation system. She recently authored a book, "Art In the Stations," with photographer Balthazar Korab.

At the same time, the endlessly energetic Walt raised funds for the more than 100 paintings, watercolors and sculptures that today grace the Alexander J. Walt Breast Cancer Center (named for her husband) at the Karmanos Cancer Institute in Detroit.

Make no mistake: The renowned art collections at Detroit Receiving Hospital and the Detroit Medical Center have played a major role in making Mrs. Walt nationally known on public art in recent years. Along the way, this champion of Michigan artists and medical patients alike received service awards from the American Institute of Architects, the City of Detroit, the People Mover and the Wayne State University School of Medicine.

Selected as "Michiganian of the Year" in 1987 by *The Detroit News*, Irene Walt long ago became a legend in her own time. For her efforts, she was awarded an honorary degree in Humane Letters from Wayne State University. She says she has "no intention of retiring," and that she intends to go right on doing her best to beautify public spaces with art.

"Money was tight, and it wasn't easy, But I found that I often got good results, whenever I told a Michigan business executive, 'Nothing is too good for our patients and our staff.'"

- Irene Walt

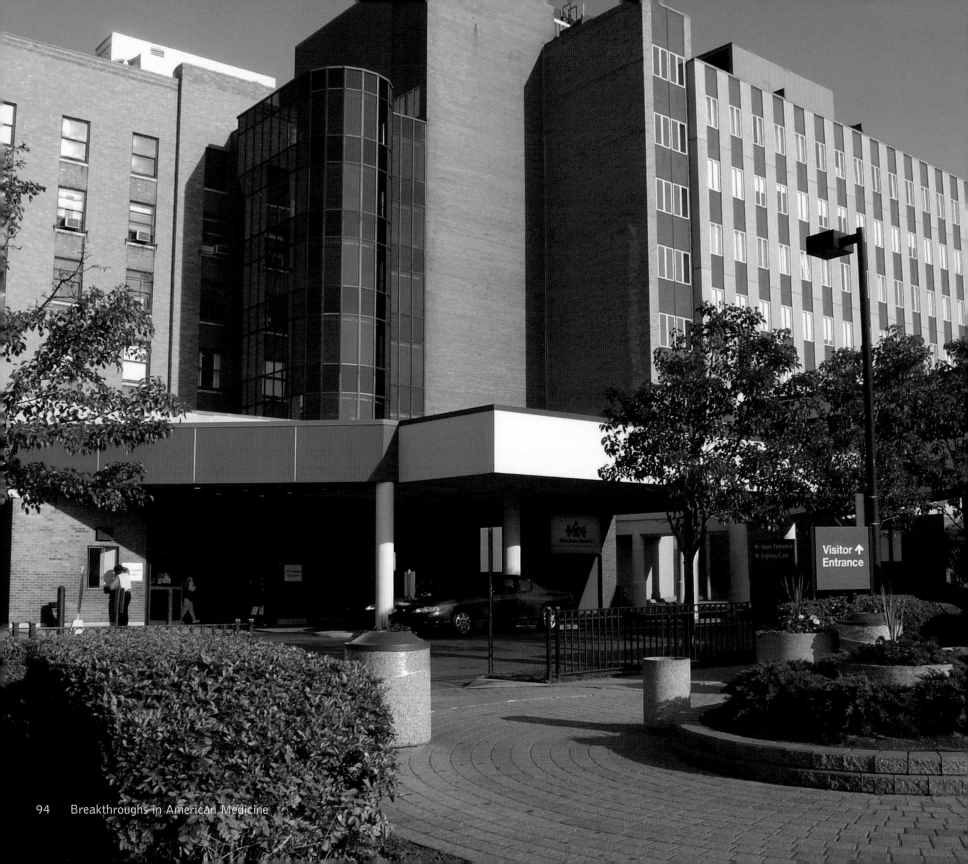

Jewish Fund donates $27 million to improve Detroit health care

Midnight. Siren howling and warning lights flashing, the red-painted ambulance zooms along Outer Drive then flashes beneath an illuminated sign:

Emergency Department.

Inside the lurching ambulance, a 52-year-old city resident is fighting for his life. Already hooked up to a state-of-the-art "defibrillator" by the Emergency Medical Technicians aboard the speeding vehicle, this heart attack victim will need every bit of the advanced medical technology and expertise available today if he's to survive this critical hour and then return to good health.

Fortunately for the patient on this balmy night in August of 2005, the ambulance is taking him to a medical facility with a reputation for outstanding emergency and cardiac care. Located in northwest Detroit, Sinai-Grace Hospital has won numerous awards in recent years for providing state-of-the-art emergency care for heart-attack patients who are treated first in the Emergency Department and then in a specially designed cardiac care facility where the latest high-tech, intensive-care tools are kept in a state of perpetual readiness.

All of this means, thankfully, that tonight's outcome will be a positive one. Having been medically stabilized and with his heartbeat now under firm control, this heart attack patient will, in the days ahead, undergo an extensive education and therapy program aimed at helping him to establish a new, healthier

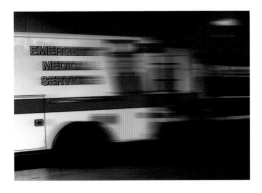

lifestyle, the first step on the road to recovery and better heart health in general.

Although our midnight patient doesn't realize it yet, his dramatic rescue and healthier future have also benefited from some far-sighted planning by one of Michigan's most effective philanthropic organizations, the Jewish Fund.

Established in 1996 with proceeds from the sale of Sinai Hospital to the DMC, the Jewish Fund has since donated more than $27 million in grants designed to expand and improve health and human services to Detroit-area residents.

Among those carefully distributed grants was a special award in 2005 of more than $800,000, a large portion of which went directly to improving both cardiac care and emergency services at Sinai-Grace. Says DMC President and CEO Michael Duggan, while acknowledging the "vital importance" of these and other Jewish Fund contributions to hospitals throughout the DMC system: "I don't think there's any doubt that charitable giving forms the backbone for many of our most successful clinical and research programs at the DMC. Nor is there any question but that the Jewish Fund has been an extremely valuable partner in the quest to provide Detroiters and Michiganders alike with the very best medical care available in the world today."

Legendary "Dr. Vee" spent 50 years developing one of nation's most admired cancer programs

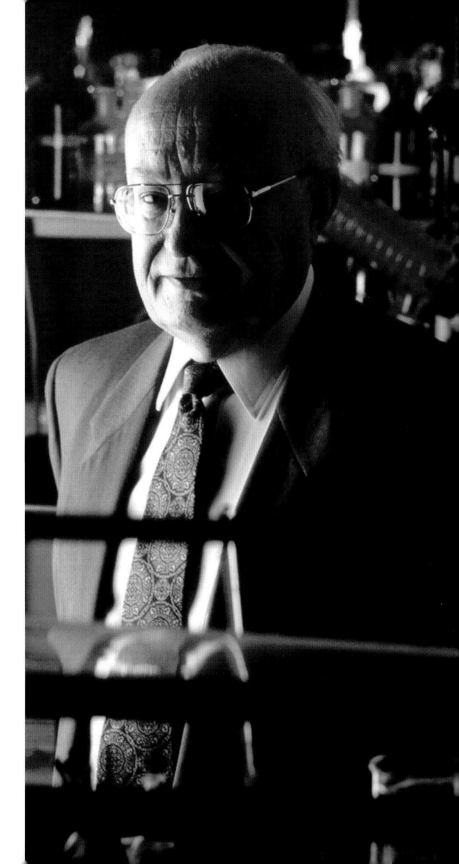

He was — and is — a legend in his own time.

He was — and is — the guiding spirit behind a remarkable oncology center that today enjoys a world-class reputation for the treatment of many different types of cancer.

Although he retired (at the tender age of 80) from his "emeritus" post as Chief of Oncology at the DMC in the summer of 2005, Dr. Vainutis K. Vaitkevicius will surely continue to make his presence felt at the midtown Detroit medical complex for many years to come.

And why not? During five decades of fiercely dedicated service, "Dr. Vee" (as he was affectionately known to thousands of patients and medical students through the years) became nothing less than an icon of the DMC whose passion for serving the needs of cancer patients never seemed to flag.

Ask any of the surgeons and physicians who have worked at the DMC during the past 20 years to describe Dr. Vee, and the odds are high that you'll find yourself listening to a reverent speech about a doctor who came to work early and always went home late — and only after the very last patient of the day had been carefully treated and put to bed.

You'll also hear a lot of stories about how Dr. Vee "fought like a tiger" to build the forerunner of what is today the world-class Barbara Ann Karmanos Cancer Institute. He was able to accomplish that primarily by using his influence as president of the Michigan Cancer Foundation (during the early 1990s) to bring together the people and resources required to build an entire hospital dedicated to treating cancer and conducting research on all its forms.

Today, less than a decade after its launch on the DMC campus in midtown Detroit, the Karmanos Cancer Institute treats more than 6,000 new patients annually and operates as an independent partner with the DMC and its hospitals with an annual budget of $200 million. Operated by a staff of 1,200 clinicians, researchers, technicians and support personnel, the Institute also numbers 300 faculty members from Wayne State University's Medical School among its medical professionals.

And there's more: In the summer of 2005, the Karmanos Cancer Institute announced plans to spend more than $70 million to expand services in southeast Michigan and all across the Midwest. That plan called for a $50 million upgrade of the Institute's main treatment facility on the DMC campus and a $3 million addition to its Lawrence and Idell Weisberg Cancer Treatment Center in suburban Farmington Hills.

The Institute also recently announced plans for two new regional cancer centers that will be located in Oakland and Monroe counties. They will cost up to $10 million each.

According to many Detroit-area medical professionals, the lion's share of the credit for the recent building boom at Karmanos clearly belongs to the indefatigable Dr. Vaitkevicius.

"There's no doubt that Dr. Vee has been and continues to be a marvelous symbol of what the DMC is all about," says DMC President and CEO Michael Duggan. "One of the first things you learn about when you go to work on the DMC campus is the power of Dr. Vee's presence throughout this entire institution.

"As a professor at Wayne State University, Dr. Vee was unexcelled. As an administrator, he left behind a permanent mark of excellence on how academic surgical departments and hospital units alike should be run in order to achieve maximum quality for patients, residents and medical students.

"His legacy is huge, and I'm quite sure it will continue to inspire all of us at the DMC in the decades ahead."

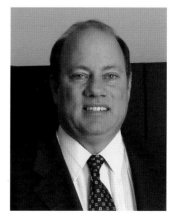

"As a professor at Wayne State University, Dr. Vee was unexcelled. As an administrator, he left behind a permanent mark of excellence on how academic surgical departments and hospital units alike should be run in order to achieve maximum quality for patients, residents and medical students."

- **Michael Duggan, DMC President & CEO**

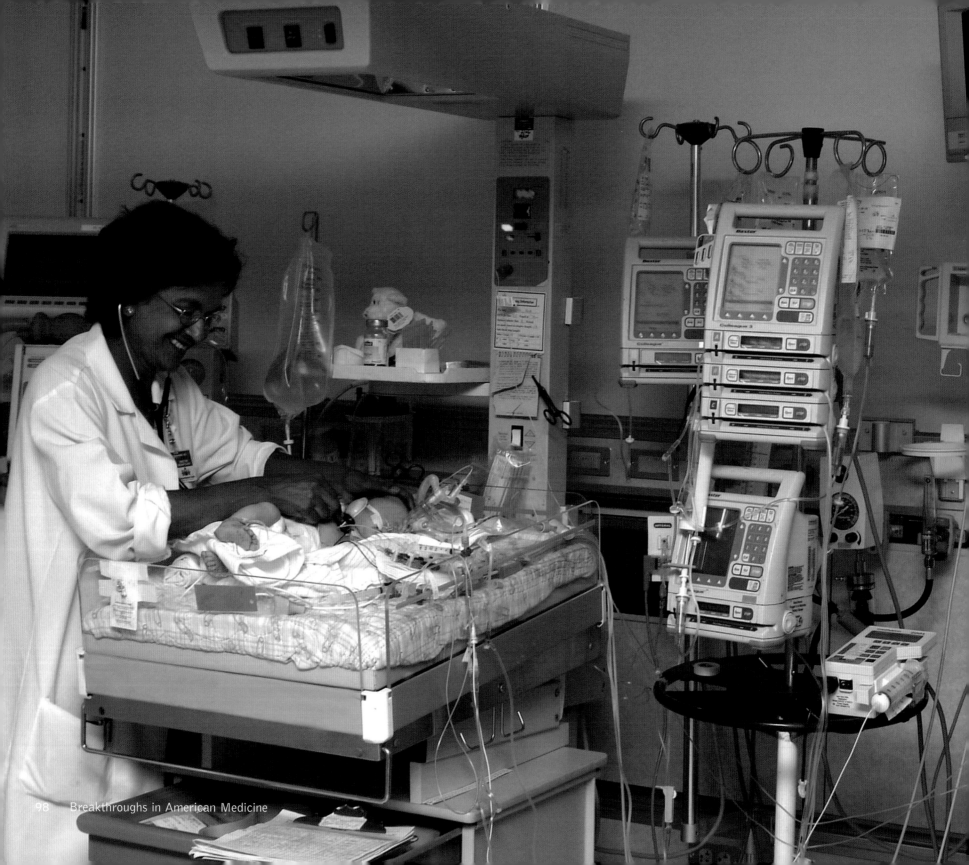

NIH funded study shows cooling babies may help prevent brain damage

Lowering an infant's body temperature to about 92° Fahrenheit within the first six hours of life reduces the chances for disability and death among infants who failed to receive enough oxygen or blood to the brain during birth. The research study findings appeared in the Oct. 13, 2005 edition of the *New England Journal of Medicine*.

The study involving 208 infants was led by Seetha Shankaran, M.D., Wayne State University Professor of Pediatrics and Division Director of Neonatal-Perinatal Medicine at Children's Hospital of Michigan and Hutzel Women's Hospital. The research was conducted across the county through the 16-site Neonatal Research Network (NRN), part of the National Institute of Child Health and Human Development (NICHD).

"This is the first treatment that we have to reduce the brain injury in these children," Dr. Shankaran said.

During the study, researchers randomly enrolled qualifying infants from the NICHD neonatal sites. All infants had experienced oxygen deprivation during the birth process. Children's Hospital of Michigan and Hutzel Women's Hospital, combined, contributed 34 infants to the study, the most of any site.

"The experimental cooling of newborns to prevent death and injury from oxygen deprivation during birth is extremely promising," said NICHD director Duane Alexander, M.D.

Hypoxic ischemic encephalopathy (HIE) occurs when the brain fails to receive sufficient oxygen or sufficient blood before the infant is born. HIE may occur hours before birth, or, in some cases, during labor and delivery. The condition may result

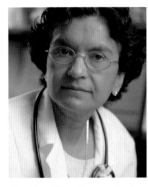

Seetha Shankaran, M.D.

from a variety of causes. These include compression of the placenta, tearing of the placenta from the uterine wall before birth, compression of the umbilical cord and rupture of the uterus.

The infants in the study were cooled by placing them on a soft plastic blanket through which water circulates. Each infant's temperature was lowered to 33.5° C (92.3° F) as measured by a temperature probe placed in each infant's esophagus. The infants in the hypothermia group were enrolled within the first six hours of birth and remained on the cooled blanket for 72 hours. After 72 hours had passed, they were gradually warmed to a normal body temperature.

When the infants were examined at 18 to 22 months of age, 44 percent from the hypothermia group developed a moderate to severe disability or had died as compared to 62 percent in the control group.

Standard care for HIE may involve placing the infant on a ventilator to assist breathing, monitoring blood pressure, providing fluids intravenously and other newborn intensive care supportive therapies.

Children's Hospital of Michigan and Hutzel Women's Hospital are the only two sites in Michigan that are currently capable of using the new treatment.

"Most newborn intensive care units probably don't have the resources to duplicate the carefully controlled conditions of the study," said Rose Higgins, M.D., program scientist for the NICHD Neonatal Research Network and an author of the study.

Sinai Guild provides funding for necessary women's screenings

Ask cancer-fighter Dr. Robert C. Burack why he can't wait to get to work each day, and this veteran primary care physician will respond by pointing to what he describes as a "very exciting" statistic: *5,500.*

That's the number of economically disadvantaged, Detroit-area women who will receive free screenings for breast and cervical cancer this year thanks to an innovative outreach program operated jointly by the DMC and Wayne State University.

For Dr. Burack, who's been running the life-saving program since 2000, that number, "5,500," holds enormous significance.

"Our cancer-screening program reaches a lot of women who might otherwise 'fall through the cracks,'" says the 57-year-old medical director of the Wayne County Breast and Cervical Cancer Control Program (BCCCP), "and that's why we're so thrilled to know that participation this year is at an all-time high.

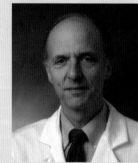

Robert C. Burack, M.D.

"There's no question that cancer screening of this kind saves lives, and our program reaches many women who are so economically disenfranchised that they couldn't afford cancer screening on their own. Our screeners often visit jails and homeless shelters, for example. But they also go into churches, department stores, utility companies and union halls on a daily basis. Nearly 75 percent of the women they test are living beneath the federal poverty line."

Although it's difficult to identify outcomes precisely in breast and cervical cancer, Dr. Burack estimates that "perhaps 40 or 50 lives" will be saved each year because of the screening program.

"As a primary care physician with long-standing interest in cancer prevention, I'm thrilled by the fact that since 2000 we've now doubled the number of annual cancer screenings we provide to women," he says. "I'm encouraged because we all know that early detection is the key to successful outcomes in breast

and cervical cancer.

"But I'm also heartened by the fact that thousands of women in the Detroit area are gaining the peace of mind that comes with learning they *don't* have cancer!"

Like most of the other doctors, nurses and technicians who staff the program, Dr. Burack is also quick to give credit to the various philanthropic organizations that help to fund his cancer-testing operation day in and day out.

One of those organizations, a passionately dedicated group of 2,500 Detroit-area women known as The Sinai Guild, has been especially active in supporting the kind of cancer screening that takes place daily at the BCCCP. In recent years, the men and women of The Sinai Guild have raised and distributed more than $1 million for research and clinical programs at all the hospitals in the DMC.

As The Sinai Guild President Rusty Rosman is quick to point out, a "sizeable chunk" of those funds has gone into major cancer-screening programs. Says the upbeat and endlessly energetic

President Rosman: "The Sinai Guild had it roots at the old Sinai Hospital in Detroit, and our organization of women goes back more than half a century. And there's no doubt that a major part of our mission has always been improving health care for *women*.

"For The Sinai Guild, cancer screening programs like Dr. Burack's are an absolute first priority."

Adds Guild Executive Director Sandra P. Jaffa: "I think the thing I like most about The Sinai Guild is that we're not based directly in any particular hospital at the DMC. That's important because it allows us to pick projects that really appeal to us. Programs like the one at the BCCCP are unquestionably saving dozens of lives each year in Detroit and that's the kind of funding project that really touches our heart strings!

"We know that many women in Detroit can't get [cancer] screenings elsewhere, and we also know that the sooner breast and cervical cancer are detected, the better the chances for a positive outcome. Really, it's a wonderful feeling to participate in that battle as a philanthropic organization."

Adds Dr. Burack, while describing the "crucial importance" of funding for cancer programs like his own: "Our goal is to reach the grassroots so we have to go where the people are. In a typical scenario, one of our [screening] recruiters will hang a [BCCCP] banner up at a local KMart or Target department store and then spend the afternoon sitting at a table, signing up women and scheduling them for a visit to a cancer-prevention clinic or maybe to one of our mobile screening vans.

"As a physician, I feel that providing this kind of screening to everyone — regardless of whether or not they have health insurance to pay for it — is a moral obligation. We have 43 million people without health insurance in this country today, and these disparities we're seeing in screening and treatment aren't going to be eliminated until we remove the economic disparities that cause them.

"Until that happens, we have to do *our* best to overcome the disparities and provide the medical care these women need. And we couldn't do it without the terrific philanthropic support we receive year in and year out."

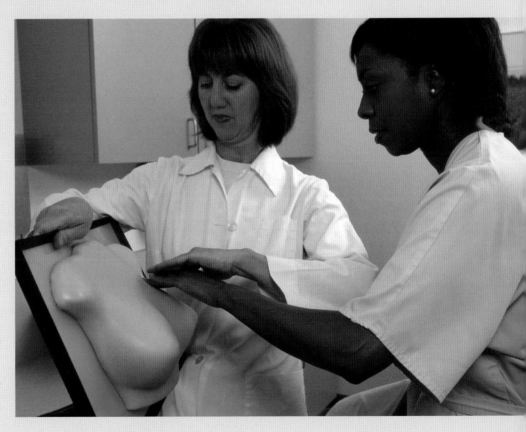

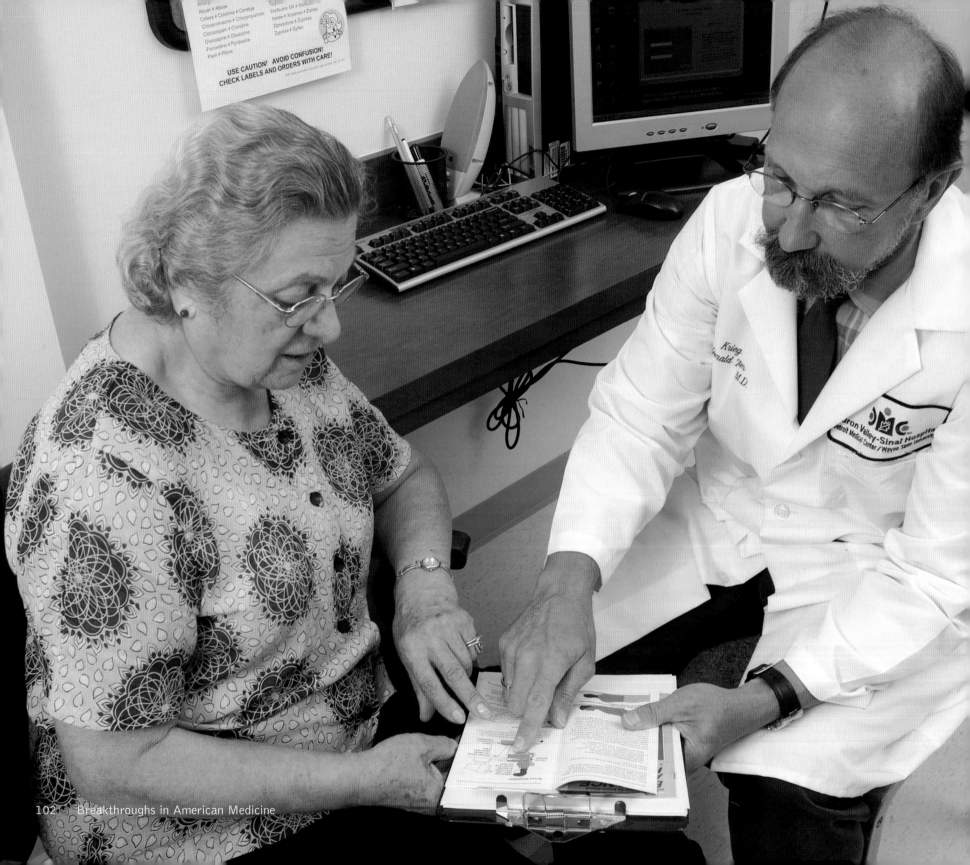

Huron Valley-Sinai triggers "inspiring contributions"

True or false: More than 75 million "Baby Boomers" will reach retirement age within the next decade, creating an unprecedented "demographic bubble" in geriatric medical care that is certain to test the U.S. health care system as never before.

If you answered "True," you're probably well aware of the huge "service challenge" that will confront geriatric health care providers during the years immediately ahead.

A troubling prospect? You bet. But one farsighted hospital in Michigan — one of the state's fastest-growing community hospitals, as a matter of fact — is already gearing up its "senior citizen" clinical and educational programs to meet the challenge.

At the DMC's award-winning Huron Valley-Sinai Hospital in western Oakland County, the highly innovative Krieger Center has launched several new state-of-the-art health care initiatives for seniors in recent years thanks to a major gift to the hospital by The Carls Foundation, which was created by the well-known Michigan industrialist, William "Bill" Carls.

Named for Bill Carls' own family physician and lifetime Huron Valley-Sinai friend, Norman N. Krieger, M.D., the thriving geriatric center takes a "proactive" approach to medical issues that accompany the process of aging. The Center provides patients with cutting-edge self-education programs, early diagnosis of age-related medical conditions and offers custom-tailored, team-oriented treatment programs. It is the only center of its kind in the area.

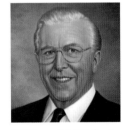

William "Bill" Carls

But the Krieger Center is just one of several highly regarded Huron Valley-Sinai Hospital programs that were made possible through the philanthropy of the late Bill Carls and his first wife Marie. Along with playing a key role in doubling the size of the hospital since its founding in 1986, The Carls Foundation contributions have continued the vision of Bill Carls "to create an outstanding community hospital."

Another recent contribution from a husband-and-wife team has established the Merle and Shirley Harris Birthing Center, which ranks as one of the Midwest's best-equipped and technically advanced maternity departments.

Another important medical breakthrough at Huron Valley-Sinai got its start on the dreadful day that Americans now simply refer to as "9/11." When Michigan philanthropists Natalie and Manny Charach arrived at the hospital to make a contribution to the cancer center on 9/11, they watched the terrorist tragedy unfold on hospital TV screens, and vowed that their gift would provide a "bright, hopeful note" on one of the darkest days in American history.

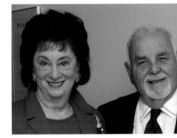

Natalie and Manny Charach

The result was the Natalie and Manny Charach Cancer Center at Huron Valley-Sinai Hospital. The Center is affiliated with The Karmanos Cancer Institute, which is designated nationally by the U.S. National Cancer Institute as one of only 39 "Comprehensive Cancer Care Centers" in the U.S.

The Huron Valley-Sinai Charach Cancer Center continues to grow and serve an expanding community that depends on its expertise and caring staff. Its very existence is an ongoing tribute to Janice Charach Epstein, who lost her own battle with cancer but whose spirit daily energizes the lifesaving clinical programs at the rapidly expanding hospital in Oakland County.

Closing in on "artificial vision"

Once upon a time, the idea that permanently blind patients might somehow learn to see again sounded like a fairy tale, like a child's bedtime story that begins with the magical phrase: *Once upon a time.*

But restoring eyesight to blind people who never expected to see again isn't a fairy tale, not any more.

It's going to happen, and soon, thanks in part to the Kresge Eye Institute's remarkable Ligon Research Center of Vision where some of the world's most advanced research on "artificial vision" is now taking place.

At the Ligon Center, a team of award-winning science investigators has spent the past several years studying how the human retina takes "pictures" of the outside world, then flashes immense amounts of image-related data along the optic nerve to special centers in the brain. These electrical-chemical "data points" are then translated into the amazingly complex phenomenon we call "eyesight."

The goal of the research is to build the first computer-based system of vision that can operate *without* depending on the eye to "see" the target and trigger the process.

Of course, the "artificial vision" project is only one of half a dozen research initiatives now unfolding at the Ligon Center,

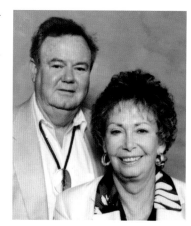

Robert and Gerry Ligon

according to Kresge Director Gary W. Abrams, M.D. "These days," says Dr. Abrams, "we've got several different teams of researchers working on issues that range from developing new 'low-vision' tools for patients with compromised eyesight to refining neural protective agents."

But Dr. Abrams is also quick to point out that the high-tech Ligon Research Center of Vision, launched back in 1998 by both Kresge and Wayne State University, wouldn't exist today without some remarkable "foresight" on the part of its major benefactor, Detroit-area entrepreneur Robert Ligon. Excited about the prospects of curing blindness in many patients, Ligon awarded a significant "no-strings-attached" cash grant to Kresge in order to encourage "open-ended research that would push the envelope and break new ground in vision-enhancement techniques."

Says Bob Ligon, while describing his motivation to fund the Center, "I've always believed that researchers and scientists should be free to follow their best impulses, based on their best understanding of the phenomena they're studying. In making my contributions to these Wayne State University and Kresge researchers, it is my fondest hope that we will be able to see the benefits within my lifetime."

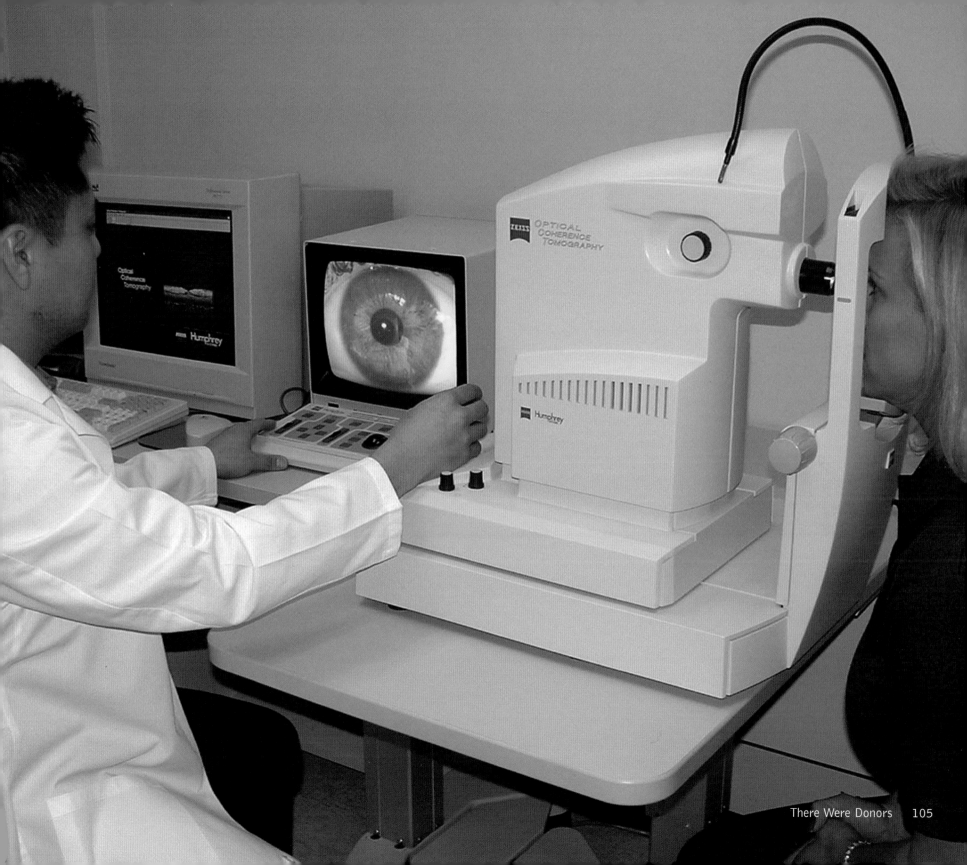

Spinal cord recovery program surges

Martin Shereda says he'll never forget the terrible moment back in the summer of 1999 when he picked up an innocent-looking telephone and then plunged headfirst into every parent's worst nightmare.

Shereda's 21-year-old son, Keith, had just been injured in a diving accident on Michigan's Lake St. Clair.

"That was a difficult phone call, to say the least," recalls Shereda Sr., a highly successful manufacturer of electrical equipment for the auto industry. "No parent ever wants to receive that kind of news, believe me. For the first couple of days, we were all totally devastated. And I could hardly bear to read the accident report, which described how my son had dived from a boat in the lake into only three feet of water.

"We sent him first to the Detroit Medical Center, and they began running tests on him immediately. Within a few hours, we knew the worst: His spinal cord was crushed, and he was almost completely paralyzed as a result. But the good news in all of this was the way that Keith responded.

"My son is a very determined, very courageous young man, and he soon announced that, in spite of his injury, he intended to make the most of his life. Quadriplegic or not, he decided to enroll at an 'online' university. I'm proud to tell you he just graduated a few weeks ago with a 3.6 [grade-point] average."

But attending college and working on an aggressive program in spinal-cord recovery was only the beginning for Keith. He was inspired by the life journey of the late Christopher Reeve, the famed "Superman" movie star who was paralyzed in a fall from a horse and then devoted himself for more than a decade to promoting research on spinal cord injuries. Keith would eventually found a philanthropic organization dedicated to the same task.

To date, the Keith Shereda Foundation has contributed more than $400,000 for research and clinical programs aimed at helping those with back and neck injuries. Says his proud father:

"What Keith did was to turn a bad situation into a positive by maintaining a good attitude.

"From the very first day of his injury, I've never heard him complain about his situation. What I *have* noticed, however, is how hard he works at raising funds and attracting other kinds of public support for spinal cord injury research. As far as I'm concerned, his story is a perfect example of how a tragic situation can be completely turned around, provided you approach it with the right attitude.

"I also think the success of Keith's foundation shows how charitable giving can have a positive impact on many different kinds of medical research. We're big fans of the 'recovery approach' taken by the Spinal Cord Center at RIM because that program emphasizes research and clinical practices designed to help patients *overcome* their injuries, rather than merely adjusting to them."

For her part, RIM president Terry Reiley says that gifts like the $350,000 the hospital received from the Keith Shereda Foundation in 2004 are "absolutely essential to accomplishing our mission in spinal cord research and clinical care."

In recent years, adds Reiley, those gifts have also included $450,000 from the Paul E. Gau Foundation and another $200,000 from the Mike Wallace Research Fund. Taken together, those monies were a key factor in the successful 2004 launch of RIM's Center for Spinal Cord Injury Recovery, which now ranks as the only rehabilitation hospital in the U.S. to focus on recovering from such injuries rather than on simply learning how to adjust to them.

"We're extremely grateful for the generous gifts designated to the Center," says the delighted RIM chief exec. "For more than 50 years, RIM has been a leader in the field of physical medicine and rehabilitation. With the addition of this new Center for SCI Recovery, we'll be able to continue our research at the forefront of cutting-edge medical advances in spinal cord injury recovery and rehabilitation while serving patients, not only regionally but nationally.

"The research now being done on spinal cord injury in areas such as stem-cell therapy is truly exciting. We hope to continue our leadership role in that effort, but we couldn't do it without the kind of support we've gotten from Keith Shereda and his wonderful family."

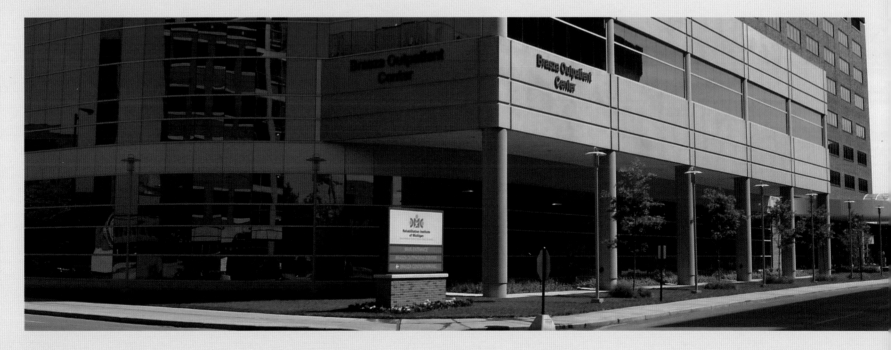

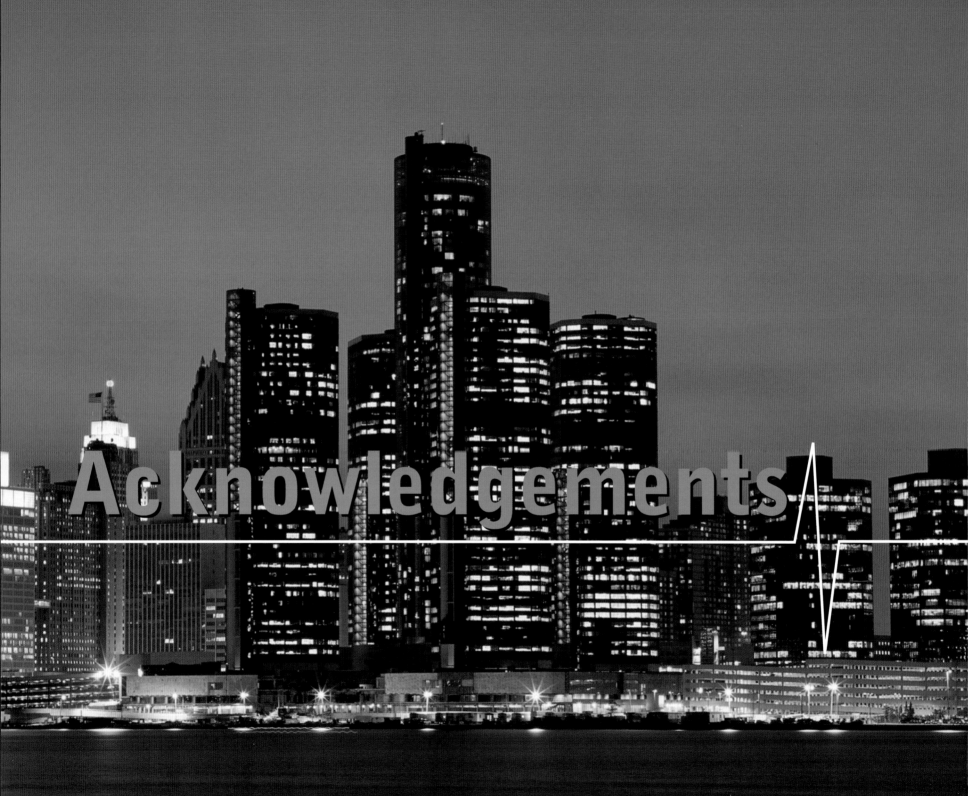

Acknowledgements

Breakthroughs in American Medicine was inspired when Robert Frank, M.D., Wayne State University School of Medicine Dean, shared at a leadership meeting the importance of promoting research that occurs on the common campus.

Nearly a year in the reporting and writing, *Breakthroughs in American Medicine* could not have been created without the thoughtful and generous assistance of many people long familiar with the history of health care in southeast Michigan. Again and again, these enthusiastic and high-spirited individuals stepped forward to provide key information and helpful suggestions aimed at ensuring the accuracy of this description of daily life on the Detroit Medical Center - Wayne State University School of Medicine combined campus.

Among the many contributions that helped to make the book possible, none loomed larger than those provided by the Editorial Review Team, which made key suggestions along the way and then scrutinized the emerging book chapter by chapter. The team included several well-known leadership figures at the DMC and the Wayne State University School of Medicine as follows:

Leslie C. Bowman, Former President, Detroit Receiving Hospital
Michael Duggan, DMC President & CEO
Dr. Larry E. Fleischmann, Chief of Surgery, Children's Hospital of Michigan
Ellen Marks, Librarian, The Wayne State University School of Medicine
Chuck O'Brien, Chairman, DMC Board of Trustees
Dr. Larry Stephenson, Cardiac Surgeon, Harper University Hospital
Dr. Iris A. Taylor, President, Detroit Receiving Hopsital

Special thanks, also, for their invaluable assistance must also go to DMC Chief Administrative Officer Richard T. Cole; to DMC Senior Vice President for Development John S. Lore; and to DMC Chief of Staff Susan Capatina.

The DMC Book Advisory Team also deserves much of the credit for making this book happen. That team included the following individuals from within the Detroit Medical Center and Wayne State University School of Medicine:

Phyllis M. Baker	**Sandy Eklund**	**Leah Ann Kleinfeldt**	**Lori Mouton**	**Douglas Bitonti Stewart**
Christine Bowen	**David Ellis**	**Richard L. Kramer**	**Maria Palleschi**	**Patricia Vinson**
Michelle Champine	**Kathy Fitzgerald**	**H. Bayard Leonard**	**Clifford Roberts**	**Juanita Wade**
Donna Dauphinais	**Leslie Fleming**	**Mary Ellen Lesperance**	**Carolyn Sabbagh**	**Cheryl Purdie Youd**
Marilyn Dow	**Bob Frank**	**Sheryl Machesky**	**Renee Shimmel**	
Daria Drobny	**Valerie Gibson**	**Bob Mack**	**Sharyl Smith**	
Cathy Eames	**Sandra Jaffa**	**Brenda Miller**	**Cathy Hall-Stephenson**	

The book was directed by Seyferth Spaulding Tennyson Inc.: Managing Editor Ginny Seyferth; directed by Brooke Vining and Julie Sabbe; creative design and layout by Joe Petz and Dan Castello; and, editing/proofreading by Karen Aylsworth.

Thanks, also, to the hundreds of DMC physicians, patients and employees who assisted in various ways over the course of the reporting and writing. Their tireless and energetic assistance was an essential ingredient in the creation of *Breakthroughs in American Medicine*.

Published by Detroit Medical Center
3990 John R
Detroit, MI 48201

Publisher's Cataloging-in-Publication Data
Breakthroughs in American Medicine. - Detroit, MI : Detroit Medical Center, 2005.

p. ; cm.
ISBN: 0-9772477-0-8
ISBN13: 978-0-9772477-0-7

1. Medicine-United States-History. 2. Medical Innovations. 3. Medicine-Practice. I. Title.

R151 .B74 2005
610/.973-dc22   2005932460

Printed in Detroit, MI
09 08 07 06 05 o 5 4 3 2 1

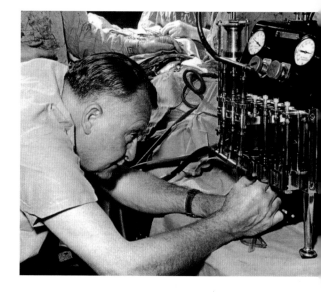